HOT✳YOGA

THE COMPLETE ILLUSTRATED GUIDE TO ALL 26 ASANAS

MARILYN BARNETT

(m)

This edition published in Great Britain in 2018 by Modern Books
An imprint of Elwin Street Productions Limited
14 Clerkenwell Green
London EC1R 0DP
www.modern-books.com

ISBN: 978-1-906761-62-2

10 9 8 7 6 5 4 3 2 1

Designer: Tracy Timson
Photographer: Mike Prior
Models: Susie Brown and Derek 'Agile' Jones
Clothing: Sweaty Betty and Bloch

Note: Whilst every effort has been made to ensure that the content of
this book is technically accurate and as sound as possible, neither the
author nor the publishers can accept responsibility for any injury or loss
sustained as a result of use of this material or any studios referred to.

This book is not authorised or endorsed by Bikram Choudhury or the Yoga
College of India.

Printed in Malaysia

CONTENTS

INTRODUCTION

Hatha yoga–the practice of *asana,* or postures–is a physical form of yoga. Essential to practicing the postures is breath control, focus and relaxation; and many physical and mental benefits accrue as a result of these. On a physical level, as the body's potential for flexibility and strength develops, circulation to the tissues is increased, bringing nourishment to more cells, stimulating the proper functioning of every body system, from the digestion to the nervous system, and increasing energy. The accelerated cellular function resulting from the process releases toxins and waste. As the body begins to function more efficiently, the better we begin to feel. The breath control and concentration each posture demands ensure that we slow down and experience our inherent calmness. All in all, after yoga practice we feel great and suddenly have a new awareness and clarity of thought. We see and respond to life differently.

There are some 80 different asanas or poses in hatha yoga, with thousands of variations. There are also many styles of yoga and schools of thought on how to practice. Hot yoga, which is described in detail on pages 12 to 15, is a practice of asanas in a heated room. One of these hot yoga styles is Bikram Method yoga, for which I am a certified teacher. This book features

my teaching of the Bikram Method style of hot yoga both in a classroom
setting and at home. The method of Bikram yoga I teach draws on my many
years' experience studying with teachers of other styles of yoga as well as
my knowledge of the human body from my medical background. This
combination has allowed me to experience incredible breakthroughs in my
postures, and I love to share this information with my students. By nature
I am an inquisitive person, and I seek solutions to obstacles. I find that the
'how to' detail offered in my hot yoga classes makes them special.
I include a detailed section on preparing the mind and body for practice.
Additionally, I suggest variations on the traditional Bikram Method postures
to make them attainable for those with less flexibility or strength.

Writing this book has been an incredible tool in exploration for me.
I will be forever grateful to the publishers for the opportunity it has given
me to go deeper into the understanding of what I love to teach.
I hope you, too, will gain in self-understanding through your hot yoga
practice.

Marilyn Barnett

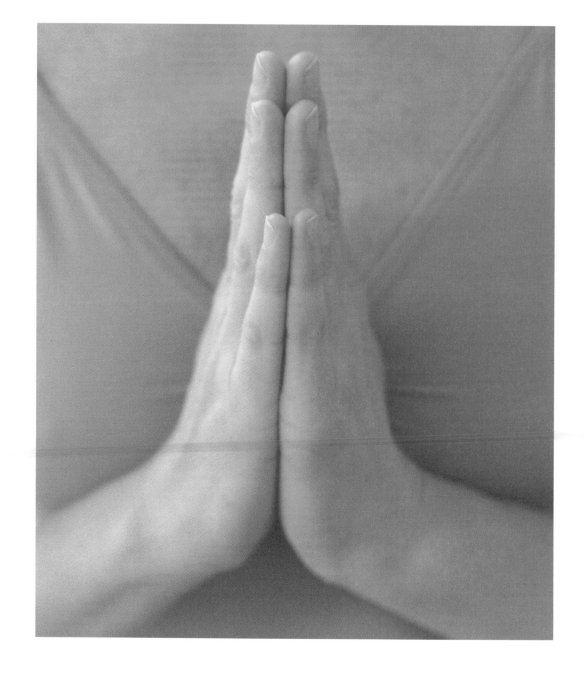

WHY HOT YOGA?

Yoga is known to restore vitality, heal and help prevent a range of common chronic ailments. Best of all, it is accessible to everyone: anyone can begin to practice yoga postures, regardless of current levels of strength or degrees of flexibility. The alchemy of hatha yoga is only augmented by practicing yoga postures in a hot room. Add heat to the environment, and along with the sweat, breath and the development of a foundation, you find the elixir of life within yourself. Heat aids the stretching process while challenging the focus of the mind, enhancing the transformational experience of yoga. When you begin devoting time to yourself through yoga practice, you find the postures and the mindful breathwork that accompanies them bring together your mind, body and soul, lifting your spirit and giving you a gift of love. Let yoga exercise your heart not with a physical workout alone, but by giving you the energy to reach out with kindness and compassion to raise the spirits of everyone around you.

WHAT IS YOGA?

Yoga is the ancient Indian science of self-discipline. The Sanskrit word *yoga* means union, and yoga practice is a path of self-exploration that unites the mind, body and spirit, enabling you to become your highest self.

The physical practice of postures and breathing that most people in the West associate with yoga is known as hatha yoga. Other forms of yoga are *karma* yoga, doing good works; *jnana* yoga, study and intellectual understanding; and *bhakti* yoga, devotion to the divine. Within hatha yoga one can practice some 80 different postures, with thousands of variations, and many schools and styles of yoga work with various combinations of these asanas.

Patanjali, a great ancient sage and founder of the science of yoga, set out in his *Yoga Sutra* (third century B.C.E.–C.E.) a recipe for attaining the state of yoga, which he defines as the cessation in the fluctuation of the mind. In his eight-fold path of yoga, physical practice of *asana*, body postures, and *pranayama,* breath control, are just two of the eight aspects (see box), cleansing and strengthening the body to enable the remaining aspects, such as concentration and meditation, on the path to self-realisation. But comprehending the theory is not enough. To understand yoga, you must practice it–with experience you think, you feel, then you know.

THE EIGHT-FOLD PATH
(eight yogic disciplines)

Yama–self-restraint from violence, lies, stealing, promiscuity and greed (the code of conduct)

Niyama–observance of cleanliness, contentment, determination, self-study and surrendering to the highest

Pranayama–controlled breathing

Asana–posture-practice

Pratyahara–withdrawal of the senses (withdrawing from objects of desire, mastery of the senses)

Dharana–concentration (focusing the mind)

Dhyana–meditation (maintaining attentiveness to the object of focus)

Samadhayah–superconsciousness (undistorted truth to nature)

Physical benefits

The physical practice of asana works on the body using contraction, stretching, compression and release of the soft tissues to create openness and evenness. These actions increase tissue circulation just as the opening of a dam sends rushing waters into smaller waterways. Areas of the body once stagnant and starting to deteriorate are flushed out by this action; they then start to receive nourishment and function fully. The increased number of cells in the body boosts the amount of energy produced while decreasing the workload on the organ systems, allowing them to perform at optimum levels, and balancing hormones and the metabolism.

Mental benefits

Yoga is an effective and efficient way to achieve physiological change, but through this process many psychological changes occur, too. Teachers of different styles of hatha yoga offer different levels of psychological and spiritual insight during class, according to their own experience and the tradition of the style. But common to all styles is the truth that when you employ breath-control and concentration in conjunction with asana, it slows the mind and induces relaxation. Overall, yoga brings a decreased resistance in the flow of energy and thoughts, leaving you free to feel, think and see from a new perspective. The transformation of your life through yoga is a direct result of this increased awareness of who you are–and what you reflect out to the world around you affects what you receive back.

Health benefits

Yoga cleans up and reconditions the pathways of physical and mental circulation and communication, bringing about positive health, hygiene and an overall sensation of well-being. This combination builds a strong constitution that helps to provide resistance and boosts immunity to disease.

Whatever the degree of physical fitness you start out from, you should adjust the intensity and level of your yoga practice according to your physical limitations, in consultation with your medical advisor and a knowledgeable instructor. For women, most teachers of hatha yoga advise avoiding very strenuous workouts in the first day or so of your menstrual period.

Yoga and pregnancy

During pregnancy, heat should be avoided in the first trimester. Thereafter, consult your midwife or doctor and a certified yoga teacher; it is thought to be safe to continue with many of the poses to which you are accustomed, but during these special months you should not begin any new yoga practices.

WHAT IS HOT YOGA?

Simply put, hot yoga is yoga performed in a heated room. Performing yoga in the heat is a practice that is becoming ever more celebrated, popularised by two main styles of hatha yoga: *Vinyasa* yoga, a flowing series of postures, and Bikram Method yoga, a set series of static asanas.

In Vinyasa yoga, the movement from the flowing sequences loosens the muscles for action and stimulates circulation. In Bikram Method yoga, the static series of postures are sequenced in a specific order to prepare the body to move deeper as the sequence progresses. The heated environment for both styles acts as a catalyst to enhance the process of relaxing the muscles as well as all of the other benefits received from working up a sweat, including detoxing the body and strengthening the heart. This book features the Bikram Method, for which I am a certified teacher.

Bikram Choudhury was the pupil of Bishnu Gosh, the founder of the Gosh College of Physical Education in Calcutta. Gosh focused on teaching physical development and mastery of a symmetrically, perfectly developed body using the science of yoga. Within this system, physical and mental strength develop simultaneously through a focus on attention and awakening the energy of willpower. Bikram was to follow in the tradition.

Aged 13, Bikram won the National India Yoga Contest, and became an accomplished athlete in cycling, running and weight lifting. Years later, when Bikram suffered a severe injury to his knee and was told he would never walk again, he returned to his teacher for help.

The healing power of yoga

Under Bishnu Cosh's strict yoga regimen, Bikram underwent a remarkable recovery within six months. With his teacher's encouragement, he began researching health benefits associated with various yoga postures. With this knowledge, he compiled a series of 26 hatha yoga postures which he adapted to address the human body's most common ailments.

The poses are practiced in a set order in a heated room in front of mirrors. After Bikram brought the method to California, it was adopted by the yoga community, spreading across the United States, Europe and Australia. Two strands of instructors now teach the style or derivations of it. Centres authorised by The Bikram Yoga

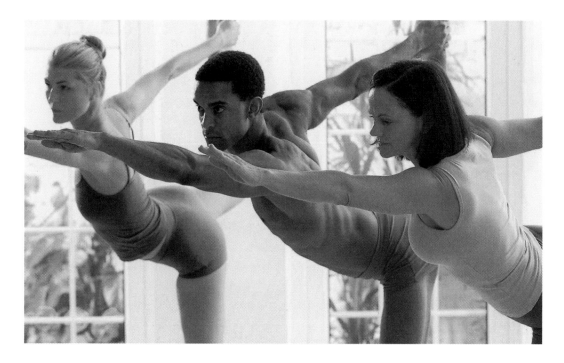

College of India offer the method in its traditional form. Other certified instructors, including former Bikram students Baron Baptiste, Jimmy Barkan and Tony Sanchez, teach their interpretations (to find a class, see page 156). In my hot yoga classes, based on the Bikram Method, I help beginners build a strong physical and mental foundation, something this method of yoga promotes well because of its static nature, repetition, mirrors and poses that work on strengthening the lower body and spine to maintain an upright posture.

Why the heat?

When your body is cold, you contract, and it becomes difficult to move. As muscles and joints warm, they loosen, decreasing resistance to movement. In a yoga class in a heated environment, there exist external and internal heat. Motion creates heat from the inside out; the heated room provides heat from the outside in, and so you move deeper into a pose with less chance of injury. 'Hot' is also a state of mind, suggestive of the intensity of effort and resulting invigoration encouraged by yoga performed in a heated environment.

THE BODY AND HEAT

Many people are drawn to hot yoga because it offers a challenging physical workout for the whole body. With application and practice, athletes, advancing yoga students and complete beginners alike can benefit from the special qualities heat brings to a workout.

A healthy body maintains a relatively narrow internal temperature range regardless of the environment it inhabits. The nervous system controls body temperature by maintaining the level of the metabolism and regulating heat loss. The largest amount of heat lost from the body results from conduction, or the flow of heat between environments from greater to lesser. By warming the environment, we can stop heat loss through conduction and facilitate the warming of the muscles and the stimulation of the circulation.

Heating the body from the inside is a result of increased metabolic activity. When it is hot, the body acts to avoid overheating and maintain healthy physiological functioning by starting to distribute the heat. It does this by increasing circulation. The heat is transferred from each cell to the fluid between the cells. This is absorbed into circulation and delivered to the surface as sweat. This form of heat loss–evaporation is the body's key way to regulate internal heat during increased heat production.

The benefits of the process

The heat-loss process at work during a hot yoga practice is stimulating and cleansing on many levels. The process of producing sweat to cool the body is a form of passive exercise because it is the reaction of the body to the internal heat accumulation that strengthens it. When the body becomes warm the hypothalamus (located in the brain) activates the body's thermo-regulation systems. The heart rate increases and blood vessels dilate to pump the warmed blood to the surface. This increase in blood flow stimulates the heart to strengthen its contractions which is exercise for the heart muscle itself. As a result, the heart pumps more efficiently thereby lowering diastolic blood pressure. In essence, the heat exposure can be a form of cardiovascular conditioning. Heat also aids in the detoxification process. Increasing blood flow also speeds up the metabolic processes of vital organs and glands, mobilising toxins for elimination. Many toxins are encapsulated in fat and stored in the body.

Heat stimulates fat receptors, activating fat stores and facilitating fat loss and releasing these fat-soluble toxins. The skin is the body's largest organ and it plays an important role in detoxifying the body.

Inducing sweat for detoxification purposes is an ancient practice in many traditions. In Ayurveda, *svedhana* (Sanskrit for sweat) is one of the five *panchakarma* or curative therapies. Additional responses of the body to heat include the stimulation of white blood cell production; boosting the immune system; promoting relaxation; and an increase in the speed of healing of connective tissue injuries and peripheral vascular disease symptoms. Overall, the body's response to heat strengthens, detoxifies and heals, which in turn creates a feeling of well-being.

Balance and efficiency

The combination of internal heat production in the presence of external heat intensifies the experience physically and mentally. Avoiding physical exertion under these conditions requires the discipline of 'balancing the opposites' while 'playing the edge', (see pages 16–17). Try to conserve energy by evenly directing and synchronising the thought (desire and attention) and breath (energy and space) on the action. Avoid struggling and find the stillness between the thoughts, the breaths and the postures. The amount and speed of movement,

the nature of the breath and the intensity of concentration all play a role in heating up a practice. Consider all of the above when setting the temperature of your practice area (see page 30). As your hot yoga practice develops, your ability to move deeper physically and mentally increases your internal heat production and the external heat can then be lowered.

Heat precautions

As humidity levels increase, the apparent temperature also increases, making you feel hotter. It is important to lower the temperature in situations of high humidity because the body's cooling system is ineffective when the sweat cannot be absorbed by the air. Adequate airflow and ventilation to the area can help to push the moisture out. Airflow is also important in the cooling process as it moves the moist air away from the surface and the new air can then absorb more sweat. Caution should be taken to avoid dehydration and overheating which can lead to heat exhaustion. Over time the body acclimatises and you become heat-conditioned; more blood is pumped to the skin, you start sweating at a lower temperature and you sweat more water and less salt. Remember that the body needs to acclimatise; if you feel symptoms of overheating, stop to cool off and rehydrate. Kneel on the mat and drink some water. Never feel pressured to continue whether in class or at home.

DEVELOPING IN MIND AND BODY

Once you make a commitment to change your life through the practice of yoga, you will find yourself developing in mind as well as body as you work through the experience. Physically, you find the strength to be flexible so that you can balance. This is mentally challenging, so you invoke self-discipline, determination and concentration to keep you going. These in turn increase your patience and give you faith, which strengthens the mind.

Physical achievements

To perform a posture, the body has to move into it. Movement occurs when one muscle shortens and its opposing muscle lengthens. The shortening is caused by contraction, which requires strength; the lengthening is a result of stretching, which requires relaxation. When both occur in equal measure, you acquire the flexibility to be comfortable within a pose. Maintaining this balance allows you to move with grace, some muscles acting as stabilisers, others providing the action. To be in perfect balance, every muscle must be able to contract and/or lengthen equally to maintain the balance of opposites as you perform a movement.

Mental growth

The process of finding physical balance challenges the mind as well as the body. First,

> ### THE PATH TO PROGRESS
>
> - Strength–being strong and relaxed
> - Flexibility–becoming comfortable
> - Balance–moving gracefully
> - Self-discipline–remaining committed to your practice
> - Determination–not giving up
> - Concentration–attending to your intention and to the details
> - Patience–a virtue that, together with all the above, gets you what you want
> - Faith–trusting the process and believing in yourself

you need the self-discipline to stay committed to your yoga practice. Second comes the determination that keeps you from giving up when you get frustrated. As you calm down, you begin to concentrate on what you are trying to bring about, and start to observe the tiny accomplishments taking place. These results boost your patience and keep you working towards your goal because you have faith in the process. And when you realise that the process worked because you made it happen by yourself, your willpower and self-esteem get a welcome boost, too.

Personal growth

Let your yoga practice be a personal growth experience. During your practice, be honest with yourself, and accept where you are in the stages of growth as you work continually to improve yourself. Obstacles inevitably present themselves. With each obstacle you encounter, pause and examine it; ask yourself what it is and why it's here right now; figure out how to move forwards while in its presence. When you understand something, you can let go of fear and resistance, relying on the process to move you through it. Finally, keep close to your heart the principles of Patanjali's eight-fold path (see page 10), set out so many hundreds of years ago. His *Yoga Sutra* contains three aphorisms that define and describe asana practice. First, keep the pose steady and firm, the mind calm and content.

Second, be aware that perfection occurs when your effort is relaxed during the extension of the mind, body and awareness. Third, it is at this point that dualities cease to exist. And so, during each posture you work on, focus on being strong, steady and calm while maintaining an even breath, and focus on the infinite; at this point, the poles of opposites are balanced. Working in this way, you stay detached from results and so move through the process of mental, physical and personal growth with greater ease.

PLAYING THE EDGE

When working through your personal imbalances, recognise your strengths and weaknesses while you maintain a balance between the two. Learn to play the edge, or push the boundary, at which comfort meets discomfort, just being there and becoming one with the action. This makes the practice enjoyable and echoes Patanjali's sutras on asana: keep calm, breathe evenly and meditate on infinity.

HOW THE BODY WORKS

To understand how your body works within yoga poses, you need some knowledge of its structure and mechanical functions. Three systems work together to allow us to move–the skeletal, muscular and nervous systems. The skeletal system (bones) provides a framework and support. Skeletal muscles attached to bones move the bones, and the nervous system communicates messages to the muscles to move, whether intentional (conscious) or habitual (unconscious).

Bones and muscles

The muscular and skeletal systems work together like a lever device, allowing a heavy load to be moved with less effort than would usually be necessary. A lever system comprises a rigid rod (here, a bone or group of stabilised bones), a fulcrum or pivot point (joint) and effort or force to move the rod (muscular contraction). Bones attach to each other by ligaments, and muscles cross these joints and are attached to bones by tendons at two or more points. The shortening (contraction) of a muscle moves the bone either towards or away from another bone, depending on the nature of the muscle action. An opposing action moves the bone back to its original position, so when one muscle contracts, its opposing muscle lengthens (stretches). Depending on the movement, several muscles may be involved, some acting as stabilisers, others providing the action. To be in perfect balance, every muscle must be able to contract and/or lengthen equally to maintain this balance of opposites as you perform a movement.

Joints, ligaments and tendons

To take a step forwards in anatomical awareness, you need to understand the function of the joints (where bone meets bone, see page 21) and in which direction movement is allowed. Bones connect to bones with ligaments; muscles connect to bone with tendons. Both are forms of fibrous connective tissue with a limited ability to stretch and contract. Stretching these tissues, especially the ligaments, results in a lack of stability to the area they support. Therefore, being perfectly aligned is very important in achieving maximum range of motion, as only when you are correctly aligned can the muscles stretch evenly. In general, the sensation of stretching should feel good; a sharp or one-pointed

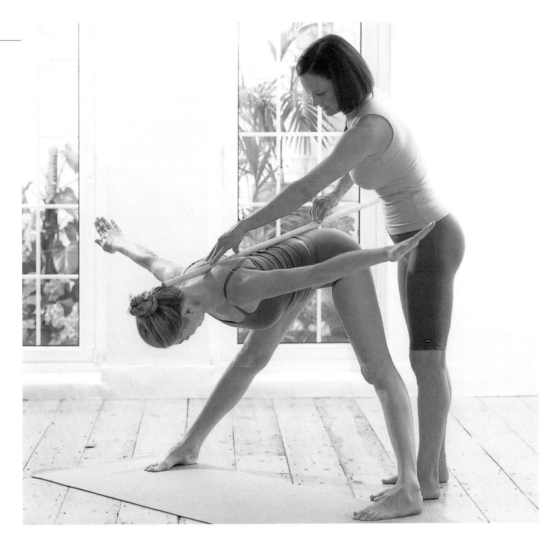

uncomfortable pulling sensation is usually a sign that your alignment is off and the tendons or ligaments are taking the strain.

Props, such as a pole or broomstick, held against the back of the body during forward bending, for example, help you isolate and experience the correct muscular movement, making you more aware of the sensation of perfect alignment in a pose.

MOVING WITH UNDERSTANDING

Unconscious muscular action–habitual patterns of movement–is the biggest obstacle to overcome in achieving correct positioning within a pose. Over the years, we each develop a unique pattern of movement: it may not be consistent with achieving a full range of motion, and it may be one-sided, creating imbalances in musculature. As we consistently initiate movements with these patterns, so we perpetuate the acquired imbalance. The key to breaking this initiation of movement is awareness.

Staying aware

Bear in mind these basics when beginning a movement. First, know the function of the primary joint involved in the action (see opposite). Second, understand the structural alignment that permits the full range of motion. Third, be aware of the effect other joints and bone alignment have on the outcome (for example, changing foot position before bending the knee alters the stretch in the hip). All this information helps you establish and maintain the best alignment in each pose to produce optimum results. Aligning the bone structure allows the muscles involved in a movement to function fully, whether they are acting as stabilisers or movers. Stabilising and developing a foundation from the bottom up and centre out communicates to the nervous systems that it is safe to move, then the muscles respond without resistance. The process of moving requires less effort when you attend to these musts. With all this to remember, it's clear why you should approach each pose with 100% awareness of where you are and where you wish to go.

GETTING TO KNOW YOUR BODY

Because of long-established patterns of movement, you may not be able to achieve perfect alignment within a posture at first. Aim to maintain the best possible alignment for you, then move to your edge. As the body responds, you will move deeper into the desired position.

JOINT MECHANICS

Spine: 33 vertebral bones divided into five segments. There is very little movement in the individual joints of the spine, but as a whole it provides flexibility to the torso that enables a variety of movements.

7 cervical vertebrae: extension and rotation. The first two vertebrae allow the 'yes' and 'no' head movement.

12 thoracic vertebrae: flexion and rotation.

5 lumbar vertebrae: extension.

5 sacral vertebrae: fused and attached to the pelvis with very strong ligaments that keep pelvis and sacrum moving as one.

4 coccyx vertebrae: fused; also known as the tailbone; no significant function.

Hip: a ball-and-socket joint, but not as flexible as the shoulder joint; allows for a wide range of movement and is very stable.

Knee: a hinge joint that allows only flexion and extension. The thigh and lower leg must be properly aligned before bending the knee to avoid weakening or injuring this joint.

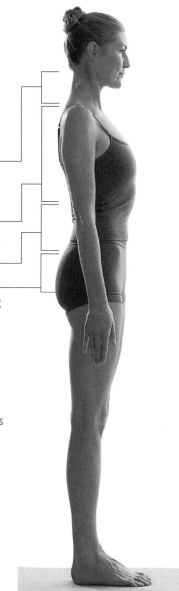

Shoulder: a ball-and-socket joint allowing flexion and extension, adduction and abduction, internal and external rotation and full rotation. It is very flexible but unstable, so be cautious when working with weight or force, especially if the supportive musculature is out of balance.

Elbow: a hinge joint for flexion and extension, and a pivot joint to allow rotation of the forearm.

Wrist and hand: the multiple bones that make up the hand and wrist provide a variety of movements. These joints are the most flexible part of the body, and their position has an effect on the joints and muscles all the way back to the centre of the body. Movement is primarily controlled by muscles in the forearm.

Ankle and foot: as in the wrist and hand, multiple bones here allow considerable movement, and their positioning has a real effect on all the joints and muscles back to the centre of the body. Movement is primarily controlled by the lower leg muscles; foot muscles play an important role in stabilising the leg.

KEY MOVEMENTS

Yoga teaches ways to establish perfect alignment in core areas of the body. Some basic joint movements are also taught in this system to enable students to achieve full flexibility.

ACQUIRING PERFECT ALIGNMENT

Stabilising the legs (below)
Press down behind the big toe, pulling in the outer ankle and side of the lower leg up to the knee; push out along the inner thigh. Pull the calves forwards and push the thighs back with the back of the knees soft (a micro-bend). Do not push back on the knees when standing upright with weight bearing down through your feet.

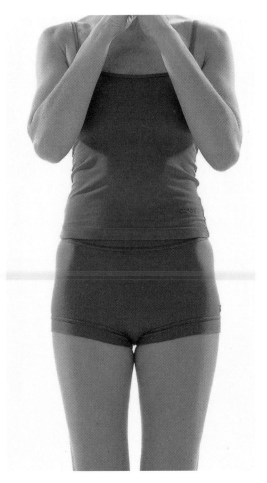

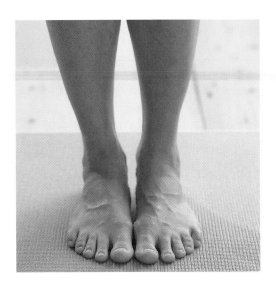

Stabilising the pelvis and spine (left)

Use the points of a diamond shape as an imaginary guide-one at the tip of the pubic bone, one opposite at the navel centre, the other two at each side of the hip crest. Stretch these points away from each other evenly, leveling out the space. Hold the space open.

After stabilising the pelvis, work with an imaginary diamond shape in the chest, stretching its points away to open the space. Find the points for the chest in the notch at the top of the sternum, at the navel centre, and just below the underarms at both sides of the rib cage. Keep the pelvic and chest diamonds open on a straight line.

Keeping the chest open (right)

Imagine the chest as an open book, its spine in the centre. Stretch from the sternum out to the side of the ribs.

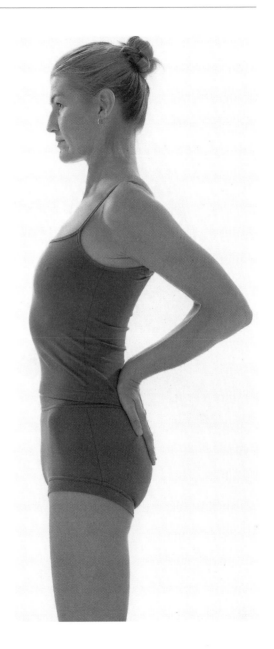

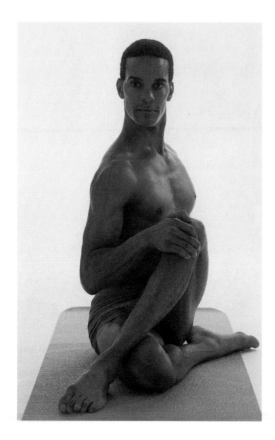

BASIC YOGA MOVEMENTS

Forward bending (below)
The hip joint is the pivot for forward bends; the pelvis pivots over the legs as the body folds in half. The spine attaches to the pelvis; lengthened and stabilised, it acts as a lever, stretching the back of the legs and pelvis as the angle closes when the two lines come together. For standing forward bends, keep your weight in the front of the feet, heels stretching down to protect the back of the knees. If necessary, bend the knees.

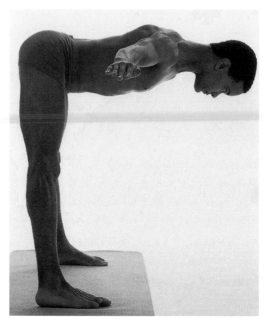

Twisting (above)
Lengthen the spine and rotate the thoracic spine to bring the shoulder in line with the opposite hip. Turn the head after completing the twist.

Backward bending (below)
Lengthen the lumbar (lower back) and cervical spine (neck) to open the curvatures in the spine, and arch back the thoracic (upper) spine. Let strength in the back of the body support the backward arc as the front of the body relaxes and opens up over it. Make sure there is no compression in either the lumbar or the cervical curvatures.

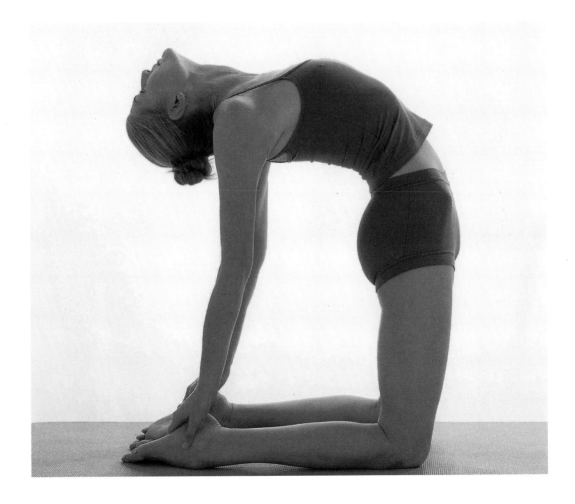

Rounding the spine forwards (below)
Lengthen the spine to open up the curvatures.
Stretch open the back of the cervical and lumbar
spine, round the thoracic spine, and lift the front
of the body against the spine to support the arc
while the back of the body stretches over it. This
is the reverse of backward bending. Make sure
the stretch to the spine is evenly distributed
along its entire length.

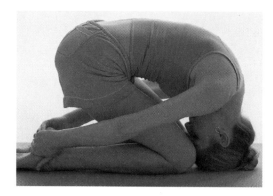

Side bending (right)
When arching the spine to the side, keep the
hips and shoulders squared, ears over shoulders.
Stabilise the pelvis and lengthen the spine, lifting
and twisting through the thoracic spine as it arcs
to one side. Lift along the side to support the arc;
stretch evenly between hip and shoulder.

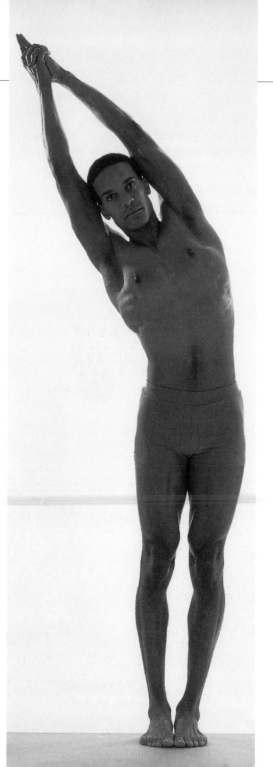

Sitting-up (below)

To perform a sit-up from lying on your back, inhale your arms overhead. Exhaling, tighten your seat and flex your feet. Keeping the legs and buttocks strong, firm your abdominals and inhale steadily while raising your arms past your ears to shoulder level. At the same time, lift your head and spine up to sitting. Exhale your pelvis over your legs. Inhale and open the spine into the front of the body. Exhale and take the spine forward from the groin up.

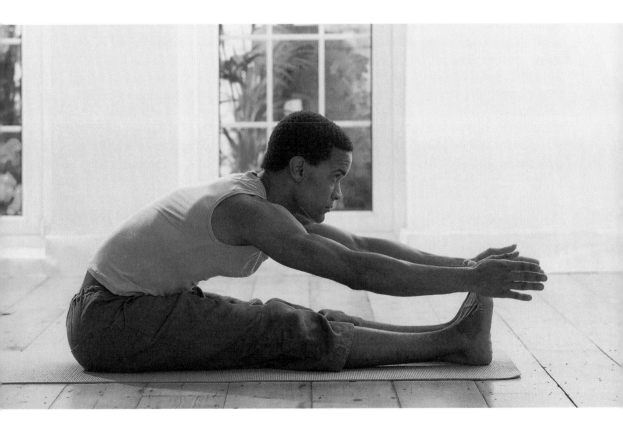

TROUBLESHOOTING COMMON PROBLEMS

Uneven use of the body

Repetitive one-sided moves or overuse of one area create an uneven musculature; if you remain unaware of this, the body continues with the pattern, strengthening it.

What you can do: Examine yourself carefully in neutral before beginning a pose. Correct your alignment, finding your centre by leveling the body, then set up a good foundation, keeping right and left sides of the spine even. Maintain full awareness as you move, paying attention to the base of your foundation: go down into the foundation before moving steadily up and out. Remember that the pose forever changes as the body develops.

Faulty foot alignment

Correct foot and ankle positioning is vital to establish the alignment that provides maximum range of motion in the joints. Overstretching the outer ankle creates an imbalance in the outer lower and inner upper leg. Repetitive action perpetuates this imbalance and limits flexion and extension of the ankle, knee and hip joints. When sitting on the heels, the inside edges of the feet should touch, fully extending the foot and lower leg. When the heels drop to the side to avoid this stretch, the outer ankle stretches.

What you can do: If the front of the ankle is really tight, support it with a rolled towel or mat, so your bodyweight does not overstress the joint. Or try this hands and knees maneuver: stretch one leg back, pull the ankle in and point all five toes evenly away from the front of the knee, heel aligned with the back of the knee. Hold, make a slight internal rotation of the leg, then, bending the knee, bring it down beneath the hip, lower leg and top of the foot resting on the floor. Repeat with the other leg, then sit back on the heels, legs folded comfortably together.

Over-stretching isolated segments of spine

This is an issue in forward bends when the spine remains unstabilised and the top of the body begins to drop below the line of the fold. The problem also occurs in forehead to knee poses where the spine rounds forwards.

What you can do: Forward bending is all about hip flexion: the pelvis rotates or pivots forwards into the thighs, stretching the back of the thighs and buttocks. The hip joint is the pivot point; the spine is attached to the pelvis and, when stabilised, works with the pelvis like a lever to stretch the muscles required for full hip flexion. Once the spine rounds forwards, you lose that stretch; stretching occurs in the rounding spine. To stretch the spine over the legs, work on pelvic flexion and spinal extension. Beware of trying to pull a rounded back over the legs: this tugs at the spine instead of pulling the pelvis forwards into the thighs. In forehead to knee poses, focus on arching the spine evenly over the femur (thighbone). Lengthen the cervical and lumbar spine prior to flexion to avoid overstretching areas of the spine at which the curvature changes direction.

Compressing the neck and lower back

Comfortable backward bending requires full extension then hyper-extension of the chest and hips: the spine lengthens and arches back, opening the front of the body. Compressing the cervical and lumbar spine prevents full extension, so pressure or pinching here is a warning to correct your position.

Dropping the head back before lengthening the cervical spine and lifting the thoracic spine into the chest strains the neck and may increase cervical compression. The weight of the head pulls the top of the spine down, making it difficult, if not impossible, to lift the thoracic spine. Depending on the pose, it can increase lumbar compression, too.

What you can do: Full backward bending is not needed for the postures in this book, but being aware of its anatomy helps you approach the poses that lead up to it. In the full backbend, the body arches back between hands and feet: the pelvis drops, making the tailbone the highest point of the spine, and the sacrum and thoracic spine lift as the spine continues to lengthen between arms and legs.

To ensure comfort while extending the spine, do not tilt the pelvis forwards; this only increases lumbar compression because the sacrum is attached to the pelvis, and to bring the spine up and back without opening the hips causes the lumbar spine to bend back sharply. When dropping the head to look up, or releasing it back during deeper backbends, bring the chin away from the throat, and shoulders away from the ears rather than bending the neck.

Scrunching shoulders

Tightness in the neck and shoulders is common when a rounded back causes the muscles that hold the spine upright to overstretch: the imbalance in the chest and back affects the shoulders and arms. When the arms rise, the shoulders move towards the ears, and stretching is felt in the side of the ribs. Holding the arms up increases the tension and becomes uncomfortable.

What you can do: Open the chest from sternum to sides, ears over shoulders, chin in neutral. Lengthen the arms by the sides, palms in; relax the shoulders down while bringing the forearms towards the sides, and straighten the arms before rotating them away from the body. Inhale, raise the forearms, exhale, relax the shoulders, and lengthen the neck and arms. Continue until the arms are over the shoulders. Bring the forearms in, palms lightly touching.

Try also a full 'yes' and 'no' movement to flex and extend the cervical spine and boost thoracic and cervical rotation. Open the chest and lengthen the arms as above. Then inhale the chin towards the throat, lifting under the ears and into the notch at the base of the skull. Exhale, relaxing the shoulders while straightening the arms. Inhale the chin to neutral, and exhale, relaxing the shoulders while lengthening the neck under the ears. Repeat, extending into the base of the skull while lifting beneath the chin to stretch the throat. Inhale the chin to neutral, and exhale, relaxing the shoulders while lengthening the neck as before. Inhale, rotating the head over the right shoulder, exhale to centre, then repeat to the left.

HOT YOGA AT HOME

When beginning yoga, take classes with a qualified instructor to get familiar with your body and movement patterns while under a watchful eye. Then use the information in this book to increase your understanding of the biomechanics of each posture, applying this knowledge to your practice. Once you feel comfortable and have a basic sense of the postures, set up a home workout space to explore the detail of each pose at your own pace.

The space

Find a quiet place free from distractions with access to heating and a well-positioned mirror. Think about the type of flooring: padded carpet challenges your stability and makes it difficult to balance in one-legged standing poses.

Heating

A radiant space heater provides the best localised heat, since objects near it absorb heat-waves. Air-blowing heaters suffice to heat an area that can be closed off to contain the heat. Heat your space to 100˚F (37.8˚C). Take care when working out in a warm environment, and monitor yourself to avoid overheating.

Mirror view

Full mirror visibility is ideal, but you may need to compromise because of expense and space limitations. The more you can see in a mirror without moving your head, the better for checking your alignment. To view every yoga position would require a mirror as high and wide as you are tall with arms overhead. However, as the poses in this book include only one posture that requires a full-width view, feel free to compromise with a near shoulder-width view in a framed portable mirror. Once you establish the sensual perception of correct alignment, the mirror becomes less important.

Yoga mat

Mats come in various thicknesses; standing and balancing on a thick, spongy mat during hot yoga can be difficult, and sweaty feet slide on a shiny mat. I find a 6 mm (1/4-inch) mat comfortable for all postures; the 3 mm (1/8-inch) mat may not provide enough cushioning for poses on the knees, back or abdomen unless the floor is carpeted. Some mats have a smooth, shiny surface; others are dull and rough-looking. Rough-textured mats are not easy to find, but are best for sweat yoga. Alternatively, place towels or an absorbent pad on your mat.

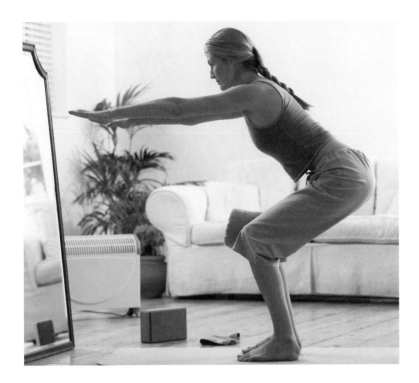

During home practice and when taking part in a timed class, keep props close at hand. Move the mat according to the instructions given at the start of each pose to gain the best mirror view for each posture.

Clothing

Besides being comfortable and allowing full range of motion, your clothing must reveal the shape of your body for visual monitoring of alignment. Stretchy, fitted garments are best. If you are uncomfortable in this type of workout wear, choose shorts so that at least your foot to knee alignment is visible. A sports bra is ideal for women; many men choose not to wear a shirt. Most important is to feel comfortable physically and mentally. For class, keep in mind that teachers can't correct what they cannot see.

Towel and washcloth

Keep a towel or two handy to place over your mat for safety and hygiene. Using a towel to absorb moisture keeps your mat cleaner and helps prevent slipping. Place a clean towel at the top of the mat during floor postures as a barrier for your face. Unique to hot yoga, washcloths prevent the hand and feet slipping in foot-holding postures. Some people just blot the hands and feet; others hold the cloth between the hand and foot. Do away with it as you develop in the pose and no longer need to grip.

Water

Hydration is essential for peak physical and mental performance. Make sure you are well hydrated before beginning practice, and keep water or an electrolyte drink available to replace fluid lost in sweating.

Hot props

Props help you progress in a pose by providing support or creating a physical environment that allows only the correct action for developing the posture. Foam blocks and folded or rolled blankets, towels, or even washcloths make good support props, raising your foundation to meet your inflexibility. They can be placed, for example, in front of the ankles when kneeling, behind the head when lying supine, or used to extend the arms in standing forward bends, taking pressure off the inflexible area and allowing the body to maintain alignment. Strength and flexibility develop evenly once the body is fully grounded into such a foundation. Select your prop according to your level of inflexibility or misalignment; as you develop, decrease the height of the prop, and eventually eliminate it.

Props are also a great way to isolate movement when learning how to approach a posture; a wall, door, pole, or blocks offer something to stabilise against, allowing you to move in the direction of the posture using contraction and relaxation. You might, for example, stand against

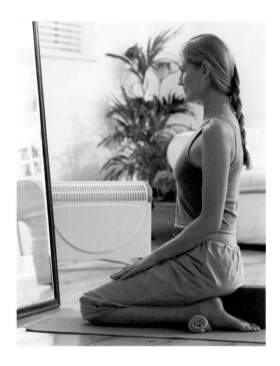

Foam blocks make good support tools. Here, they allow the body to remain aligned in the pose. A rolled washcloth takes pressure off the ankles.

a wall to establish proper front-to-back alignment, or try forward bending with a pole held against your back. To reinforce standing upright, try standing facing the narrow edge of an open door with feet on either side of the door beneath the hips. Bring the spine forwards to hold the front of the body up against the door edge. Using props in this way is best confined to self-exploration or private lessons.

PREPARING FOR PRACTICE

Yoga practice offers valuable time to spend with yourself that enhances your physical, mental and spiritual qualities. Being prepared makes the journey that much more enjoyable and effective. Plan ahead by setting aside adequate time and preparing yourself physically and mentally; you will then be able to focus fully on your intentions when it is time to begin.

PREPRACTICE RITUALS

• Be hydrated: drink plenty of water throughout the day. Excessive amounts of liquid just before class may not be comfortable and you may need to disrupt your practice to relieve yourself.

• Don't eat a heavy meal within two hours of practice: the stomach should be empty for yoga. If you do need to eat, choose easily digestible food.

• Take a hot bath if you feel stiff or need relaxing.

• Centre yourself: take a few moments to be still and feel your breath, allowing yourself just to be.

• Mentally dedicate your practice to yourself.

When you start your practice, work through every pose efficiently, playing each edge as if you will be in the pose forever. In this way, yoga becomes a meditation in motion and you find yourself contemplating the infinite. This gradual process is effective in helping you develop each movement from the bottom up and the inside out; and so you build a solid pose.

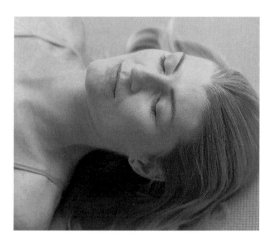

Working with the breath

Use your breath to help you work through the postures, mindfully synchronising it with the thought, feeling and action of the move. Breathe in through the nose and out through the mouth, using the throat to control the volume and mentally directing the flow of air through the body. With each inhalation, draw strength in from your foundation and take space to restricted areas. As you exhale, stabilise your foundation and relax tension around newly created space, moving deeper in the direction of the desired pose.

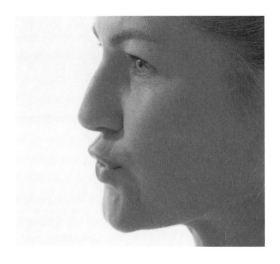

Setting up for breathing

Softly close your lips and use your throat to monitor the flow of breath, drawing it in slowly and evenly, and filling the lungs fully from bottom to top. Then open your mouth and let the breath out with the same control, emptying the lungs completely. The breath is audible: when you inhale it is a high-pitched 'HUMMMMM;' the exhalation sounds like a low-pitched 'HAAAAA.' Treat the inhalation and exhalation as separate actions, completing each one before beginning the next. Make the transition between them smooth so that you don't begin with a quick rush of air. This would cause the top portion only of the lungs to fill or empty, making it difficult to complete the action. If you have problems controlling the flow of breath, work on evenness, making sure you

don't gasp in or expel out too much air at once. In the first pose (pages 40–43), work up to a full six-second intake and expelling of breath, keeping it even from the very beginning to the end in each direction. As the capacity of your lungs increases, resistance decreases and you will be able to move more air during the 6 seconds.

TADASANA

To begin your yoga practice and between each standing posture you adopt a basic standing pose known as Tadasana or Samasthiti. The feet stand parallel to each other (as shown opposite) and all the joints are aligned so that the body remains in line from ears to ankles through the centre of the joints. The eyes, shoulders and hips stay level.

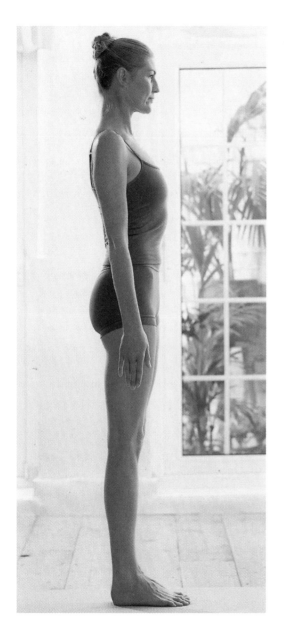

Setting up for Tadasana

Place your feet parallel to each other: visualise a line from the base of each second toe to the centre of the ankle on each foot and place them parallel. Bring the knuckles of the big toes to touch and place your heels directly behind your toes. Lift your toes, stretch the ball of the foot wide and press down into the floor. Relax the toes lightly on the floor while keeping your weight evenly distributed between the sides of the heels and the balls of the feet, which anchor to the floor.

Take your thighs back so the hips are directly over the heels, knees centred between hip and ankle; there should be a softness or microbend behind the knee.

Square up your pelvis and shoulders (see stabilising the pelvis and spine, page 23), and bring your ears over your shoulders, chin parallel to the ground.

With arms at your sides, palms facing in, hold your chest open and draw the elbows towards the body. Stretch your palms open, then relax the arms and hands. Soften your eyes and gaze straight ahead. If necessary, keep your toes up to stabilise the upright alignment. If having the knuckles of the big toes touching feels unstable or uncomfortable because the knees or thighs are too close, separate the feet slightly.

RELAXATION IN
SAVASANA

Dead Body Pose, Savasana, is the finishing touch to your practice and one of the most important poses to follow any yoga routine. You will find instructions for final Savasana in a class setting on pages 152-155. At home, props such as pillows, blocks, or folded blankets can help you more readily to find the state of deep relaxation brought about by Savasana. Beginners and less flexible students especially benefit from this approach.

Savasana between postures

Savasana forms the transition between the standing and floor postures. Once you have finished Tree Pose (see pages 88-91) and have taken two breaths in Tadasana, lie back on your mat for two minutes of quick relaxation. Return to this neutral place again after each floor pose. Between the spine-strengthening postures, use a version of the pose lying on your front during the brief transition between the poses.

Using props in Savasana

Choose a light blanket or shawl to protect you from drafts; use blankets or towels as suggested:

Supporting the head

- Use a rolled blanket or towel to support the curve in your neck.

- Add support to either side of your head with rolled towels or pillows for a little extra treat.
- Cover your eyes with a soft cloth or eye pillow to aid withdrawal from the outside world.

Supporting the arms

- Place a folded towel or thin pillow beneath your forearms to support your wrists and hands and provide elevation to ease returning circulation.
- Fold a towel to make a support at least as wide as your chest and approximately 10-15 cm (4-6 inches) in length. Place it between your underarms and shoulder blades to create a slight upper-back bend that gives the chest a gentle stretch and promotes opening in the heart centre.

Supporting the legs

- Place a folded blanket or bolster beneath your knees to support them if, when you fully extend

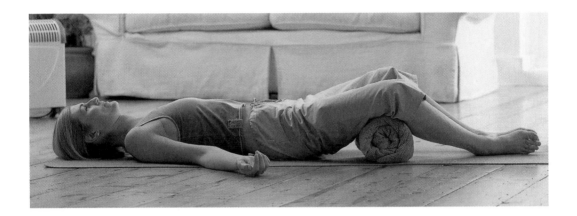

your legs, your pelvis tilts out of neutral. This removes pressure from the lower back and is promotes complete relaxation.

• Draw the soles of the feet together and up, then place supports beneath the outside of the knees and legs as they relax (shown above).

Letting go

Students of yoga use a variety of visualisation and breathwork techniques to help let go of extraneous thoughts as well as tension in the body during this final relaxation. Experiment with the suggestions here:

Using the breath

Inhale slowly from fingertips to shoulders. Roll the breath around the shoulder joints, and slowly exhale through the elbows, past the wrists and hands, and out through your fingers. Inhale slowly into your navel, draw the breath up the spine to the back of your head and slowly exhale through your face, throat, chest and out through your belly. Inhale slowly through the tips of your toes, taking the breath up your legs into your hips. Gently squeeze the buttocks, release and exhale down the legs past the knees, ankles, feet and out through your toes. Inhale again, taking the breath from the soles up through your body to your crown. Pause, and exhale very slowly through the entire body, releasing all fear, worry and tension.

Giving thanks and just being

Adopting an attitude of gratitude, breathe in and allow thanksgiving to fill you. Breathe out and feel love surrounding you. Count your blessings with each breath.

Inhale a slow, full, deep breath. Exhale a long, releasing breath and allow yourself simply to be. Practice being more and doing less.

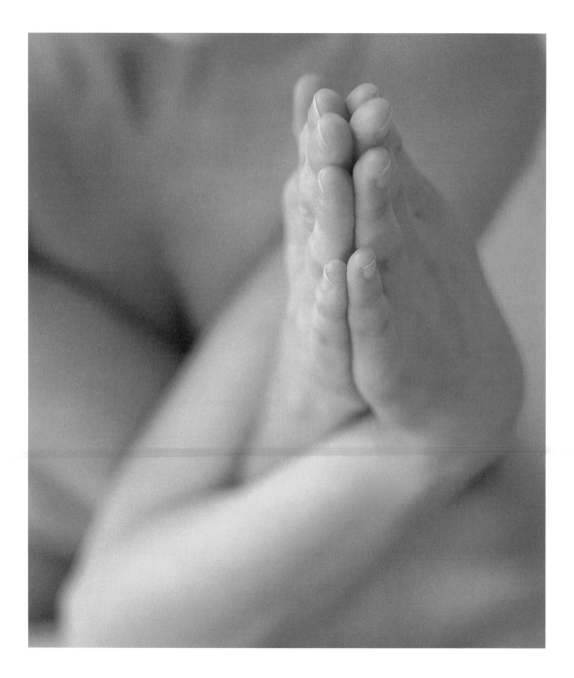

THE POSES

Within this chapter you will find instructions for poses practiced in a Bikram Method hot yoga class. We start with standing poses overleaf, and then move on to poses practiced lying or kneeling on the floor. Correctly positioning and aligning the body within each pose is of key importance, since only in this way are you able to bring about the desired response of body and mind to a particular posture. Once you begin to feel the difference between a correct and incorrect posture, you quickly become able to reposition yourself. Treat the instructions for each pose in the pages that follow, with their great detail and intense scrutiny of positioning, as a virtual teacher, consulting the hot tips to check on your alignment and movement within each stage of an asana, and to troubleshoot common problems. Be patient with yourself; this book offers a great deal of information, and assimilating it into your practice takes time. Each body is unique, and every one of us will work through many stages of development in a pose. Where necessary, I suggest alternative ways to approach a posture as you develop the balance between strength and flexibility required to perform the pose in the tradition of the style. Some of the alternatives are modifications that isolate the movement so that you use the right muscle groups. This allows you to connect with the sensation, providing a physical as well as a mental understanding of the intention behind each pose. Whatever your starting point, enjoy your practice.

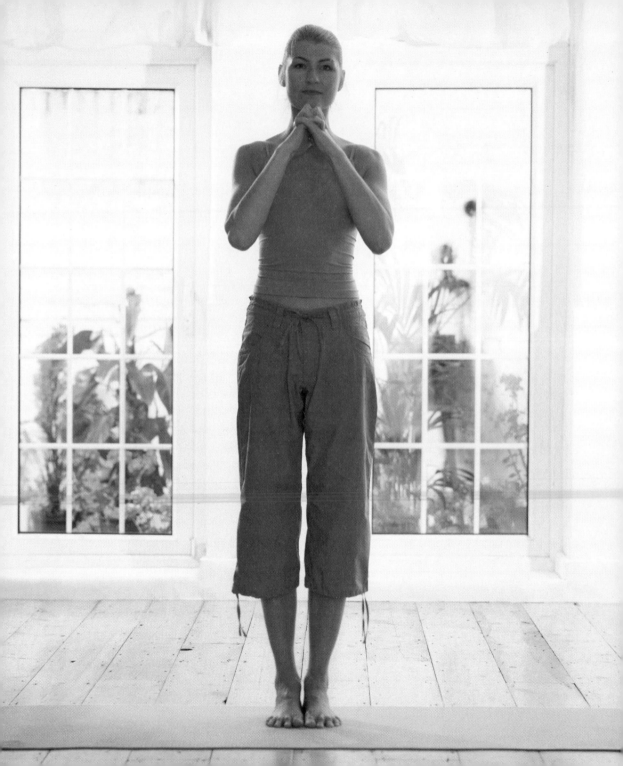

STANDING DEEP BREATHING

PRANAYAMA

Warm up with a breathing exercise (the Sanskrit word *prana* means breath or life-force) that begins to warm the body, open the airways and stimulate the lungs. As the air moves deeply in and out of the lungs, their capacity is increased. When performed correctly, the head and arm movements that accompany the breath lengthen, relax and strengthen muscles in the shoulders, arms, neck, chest and upper back while empowering the stabilising muscles of the shoulder joints. Mentally, slow and controlled breathing calms the mind and connects you with your body as you actually begin to feel yourself breathe. Beginners may find it easier to practice the breath technique on page 34 separately before putting it together with the body movements. Throughout, work on maintaining even control of the flow of breath: try not to gasp in or expel out too much air at once.

STARTING POSITION: *top of the mat towards the mirror; standing at the centre of the mat facing the mirror.*

SETTING UP From Tadasana, basic standing pose (see pages 34-35), interlace your fingers to the webbing and place your knuckles under your chin. Keep your chin down, neck in a neutral position. Point your elbows to the floor, separated to make a straight line from second knuckle to elbow. Straighten your wrists, relax your shoulders and open your chest. Gaze straight ahead. The chin and knuckles stay connected through all four movements. Try to keep your body stable and still; only your arms and head move. Use the breath technique on page 34.

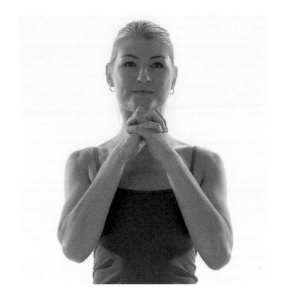

1 Arms only

Keeping your chin down, start separating your elbows and circle your arms up and in towards your ears. Keep your wrists straight, shoulders relaxed and neck long. Draw your arms down into the shoulder joints as they circle upwards, raising them as high as you can without lifting shoulders to ears. Feel the movement in your arms, shoulders and upper back, rather than as a lifting and stretching from the middle of the torso. Sense a nice opening and stretching of the palms as the elbows move towards your head.

✳ **Hot tips** Don't let the shoulders rise when you bring the arms up. Lengthen the muscles around the neck, shoulders and arms to bring the arms up closer to the ears. Initiate arm movements with the forearm bone.

2 Head only

Keeping your neck neutral and stable, lift your chin away from your throat (pivot the head up as if beginning the 'yes' head movement) to stretch the throat. Keep your knuckles and chin connected and your elbows up. Take your gaze upwards. Be careful not to crunch the back of the neck.

3 Arms only

Keeping the elbows up, bring your forearms towards each other without bending your wrists or moving your torso. Try to keep your forearms parallel with the ceiling, your body parallel with the mirror. Don't let the front of the body collapse to touch elbows.

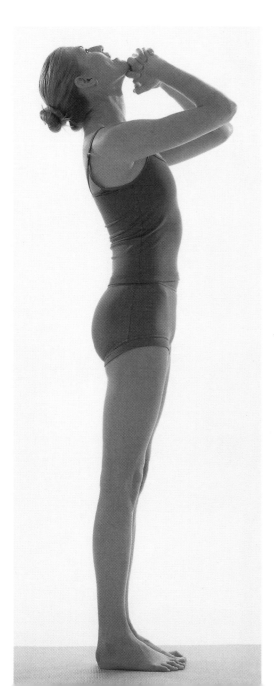

4 Head only

Bring your chin back towards your throat, elbows pointing down in the starting position. After each set of movements, return your arms to your sides, bring your chin into your throat and relax your head and shoulders down to the basic standing pose. Begin setting up again and work up to 10 cycles, ending with the fourth movement.

WORKING THE POSE When putting all the movements together, inhale during step 1, pause the breath on the transition, then complete the second step. Exhale during step 3, pause during the transition and again before completing the final step. As you become more comfortable at putting it all together and are able to maintain an awareness of the breath and movements simultaneously, make the sequence more continuous by beginning the exhalation on the second move, completing it with the third move, beginning the inhalation on the fourth move, and completing it with the first move. It goes like this–inhale, arms circle upwards; exhale, chin up and arms circle around; inhale, chin down and arms circle. Be careful not to cheat yourself of the entire range of motion you experience when completing each movement fully.

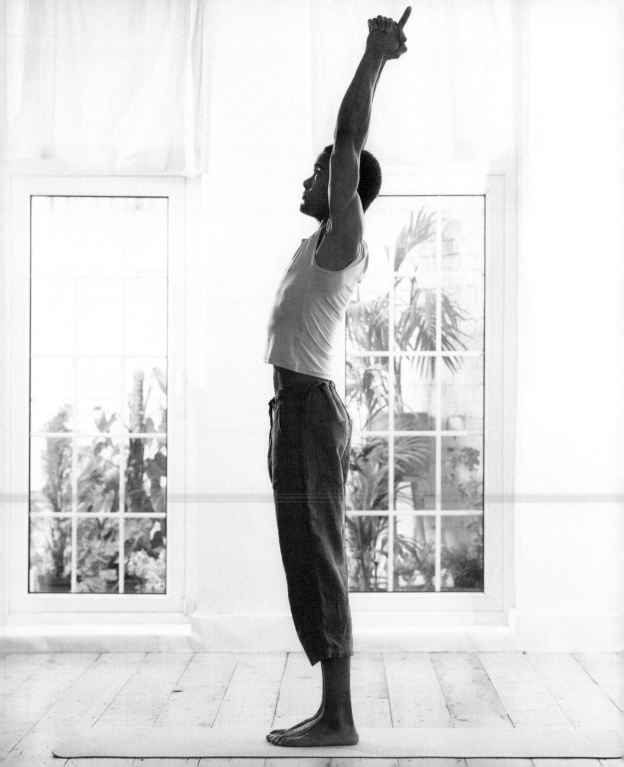

HALF-MOON POSE WITH HANDS-TO-FEET POSE

ARDHA CHANDRASANA
& PADAHASTASANA

You take on the form of a crescent moon (*ardha* means half, *chandra* moon) in this second standing pose in the series, which awakens and warms up the spine. There are four parts to the pose: by following side bends to the right and left with backward and forward bending, you strengthen and lengthen all four sides of the spine, and stretch your extremities, too. In the hands-to-feet forward bend, you gradually progress into a deep forward bend that stretches the lower spine and allows gravity to elongate the rest of the spine. It also provides a good stretch for every part of the back of the legs.

STARTING POSITION: *standing at the centre of the mat facing the mirror.*

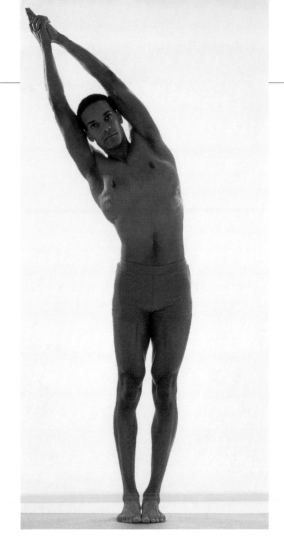

SETTING UP From Tadasana, inhale and raise your arms slowly overhead. Interlace your fingers and release the fourth fingers like a steeple. Exhale, relaxing the shoulders. Draw your elbows in, straightening the wrists and bringing your palms flat together. Do not grip the palms; gently move the forearm bones in while relaxing the shoulders. The wrists and elbows begin to straighten, the chest opens, and the upper back muscles activate to stabilise the shoulder joints and hold the chest open. Aim to stand erect, arms overhead aligned with the ears, spine in a neutral position through all four parts of the pose.

1 Right side bend

Stabilise your legs and pelvis, then lift the spine vertebra by vertebra out of the pelvis. When you get to the thorax (ribcage area), continue to lift, slightly rotating the right side forwards, left side back so the shoulders stay square with the pelvis, the chest open. Relax the shoulders away from the ears, and draw your forearms in, straightening wrist and elbow joints. From the front you resemble a crescent moon, the spine forming the arch between straight legs and arms. Feel your weight evenly distributed in the four corners of your feet. From the side, everything aligns: if standing in front of a wall, legs, hips, both shoulders, head and arms would touch it. Work with the breath for 1 minute–about 6 breath cycles. Inhale to come up, and exhale. Pause in the centre. On the next inhalation begin setting up to bend left.

Hot tips Shoulders scrunching, chest collapsing, or back arching? Set up again, then raise the arms without lifting the shoulders. Stretch up and over a few times. Return to centre and check your alignment.

2 Left side bend

Reverse the directions for step 1 to work with the left side. Let the left side of your body support your posture while the right side relaxes and lengthens. Inhale, stabilise your legs, draw strength into the left side of the spine and move it towards the centre. Draw your forearms in, maintain the lift in the centre of your torso and keep your shoulders down. Exhaling, release and lengthen between ankles and hips, hips and shoulders, and shoulders and wrists. Simultaneously stretch the right side of your body from hands to feet while strengthening the muscles that stabilise the left side of your spine. Work with your breath for 1 minute, drawing in strength and space to appropriate areas when inhaling; stabilising and relaxing into the stretch on the exhalation. Come up on an inhalation, and exhale at the centre. On the next inhalation, begin to set up for bending backward.

Hot tips Hinging from the waist or hips when folding to the side? Work on creating alignment on all four sides of the body: start from the inner ankles and sense the line up through the perineum, navel centre, heart centre, throat centre, crown of the head and along to the inside of the wrists and palms.

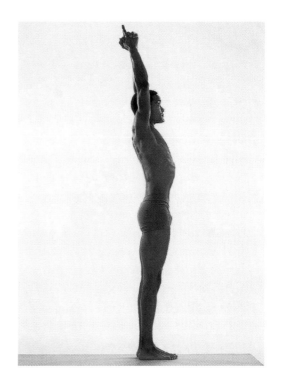

3 Backward bend

Draw the calves forwards and down, thighs back and up, stabilising the pelvis and legs (weight in heels). Release the tailbone down and spine up. Relax chin to throat, taking the arms back (head between). Lift the chest with the spine. Don't move the thighs forwards: stack leg and hip joints. Making a line from fingertips to lower shoulder blades, inhale, tailbone to heels, stabilise, and open the chest. Exhale chin to throat, head and arms back. Work for 1 minute.

4 Forward bend

Stabilise the legs (take the calves forwards, thighs back, lower legs inward, upper legs out). Begin to rotate the pelvis forwards, and, maintaining a straight line from fingertips to tailbone (chest up, as if folding in half from the top of the thighs), take your hands to the floor. Let your head hang, shaking 'yes' and 'no' to release tension. Warm up by walking out the legs-bend one knee at a time and stretch up to the hip of the straight leg. For a different stretch, lift the heel of the bent knee and bend and straighten both knees together a few times. Then, with bent knees open, flatten out the diamond in the front of the pelvis (pubis to navel, hipbone to hipbone) and place it on your thighs. There should be no space between pelvis and thighs. Reach around and place your fingers under your heels, cupping the heels, forearms on the back of the calves, elbows pointing upwards. Feel the weight in the balls of your feet, heels reaching into your palms. Let the rest of the torso relax over your legs and your head hang. Work with your breath for 1 minute.

Hot tips Can't turn the pelvis because of tightness in the back of the legs? Begin to bend the knees and allow the body to fold in behind. At the groin, bring the front of the hipbones on to the thighs, lower ribs to thighs, chest to knees, hands to the floor.

WORKING THE POSE Connect your ankle bones, outside to inside; inhale; draw your lower legs in, upper legs apart. Exhaling, move your calves forwards, thighs back. Keep the pelvis gently pressing flat on the front of the thighs and relax the torso, letting gravity lengthen the spine. Keep your forearms on the back of the calves, back of the lower legs stretching into your palms. Hold the elbows up, shoulders away from ears, crown of the head moving towards your feet. The back of the thighs stretch up to the sitting bones.

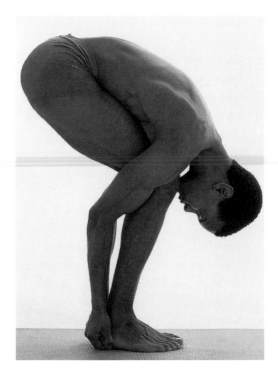

Hot tips Can't keep the pelvis on the thighs? Don't continue bending forwards. Lifting the diamond shape of the pelvis away from the thighs moves the stretch from the back of the legs, and only an isolated, weak, portion of spine stretches. Continuing to bend forwards only increases the flexibility and emphasizes weakness See the tips on forward bending on page 24.

If you are using the body unevenly, see page 28. Try also practicing the pose with feet slightly apart for better stability.

COMING OUT Inhale and lift your chest, creating a line from fingertips to tailbone to stabilise the torso, then lift your hipbones away from your thighs. Bring your body up in one piece from the hip joint (rotating the pelvis back up). In the beginning, you may need to bend your knees when lifting the chest to create a straight energy line from fingertips to tailbone. Then lift your body away from your legs and straighten your legs on the way up. Exhale and take your arms down to your sides.

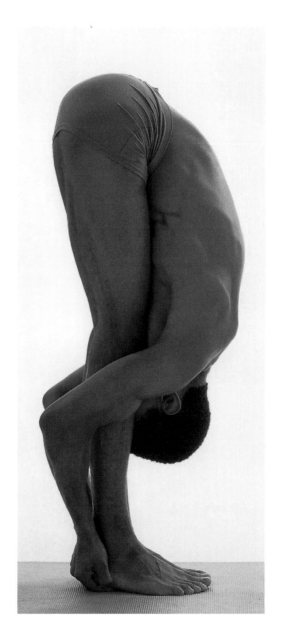

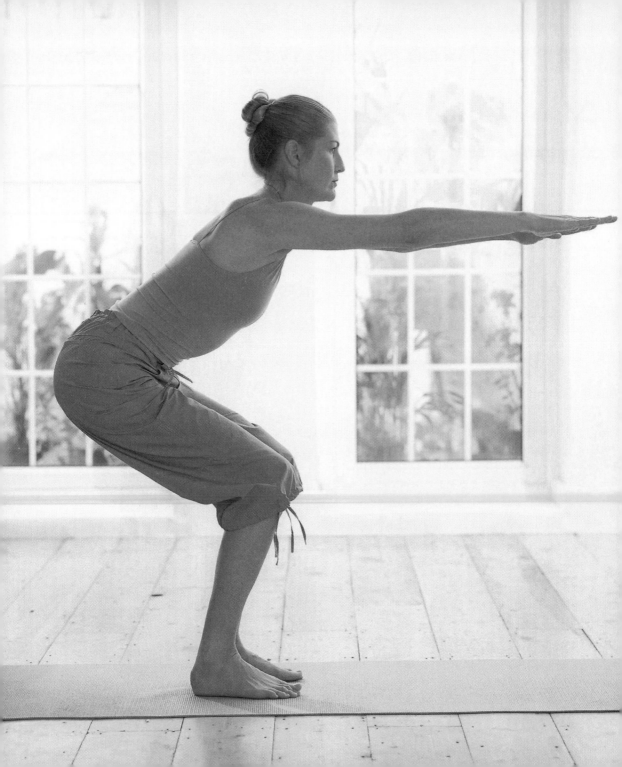

AWKWARD POSE

UTKATASANA

There are three postures within the third pose of the standing series, which warm up the lower body and the mind. Physically, these stretches work primarily on the legs, strengthening all the muscles here as well as the ankle and knee joints. They also improve core stabilisation by toning the abdominals, upper back and the arms, especially the triceps. As the name suggests–*utkata* signifies powerful or mighty–the movements as well as being awkward to master, test your focus and concentration as you try to maintain complete steadiness of mind and body.

STARTING POSITION: *standing at the centre of the mat facing the mirror.*

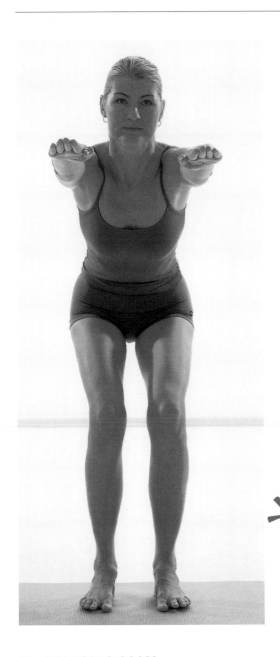

SETTING UP From Tadasana, separate your feet hip-width apart. Use your front hip bones as a guide and centre your ankles beneath them. Make sure your feet are planted directly beneath your hips so your legs and feet are aligned parallel with each other from the top of the thigh to the ankle to the base of the second toe. Use the midline of your legs, rather than the edges, as your guide. Keep your toes relaxed, resting on the floor. Inhale and raise your arms to shoulder-height. Draw your forearms in to align the arms, straight from the middle finger to the centre of the upper arm, and parallel with each other and the floor. Exhale and relax your shoulders. Keep your arms in this position through all three postures. Ensure that your ears are over your shoulders and your chin is parallel to the floor. Keep your chest and abdomen open wide and long, your stomach in and up, your shoulder blades in and down, and let the shoulders relax. Keep your gaze straight ahead and your breath smooth and even.

Hot tips Look at your feet. Too close together or too wide apart and the ankle and hip joints won't align, increasing instability.

Can't hold the arms up without tensing neck, shoulders and arms? Inhale, drawing the forearms in. Exhale, hold them up (as if heavy), and relax shoulders away from ears. This engages stabilising shoulder muscles.

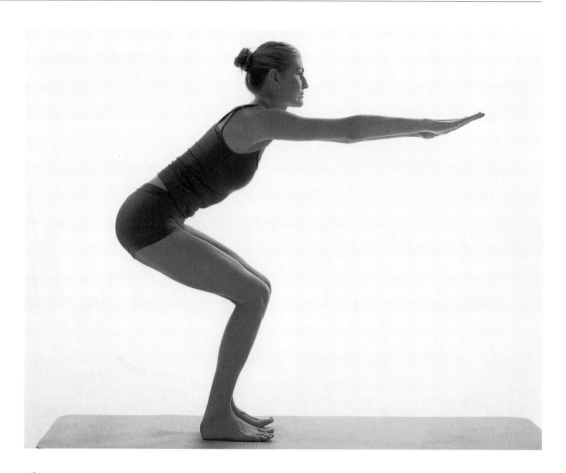

1 Fold forwards

Folding from the hips, take your body forwards and down, raising arms parallel to the floor in an upside-down 'L.' Lift all ten toes, press down beneath the big toe, then stretch across to the outer edge of the feet, both sides of the heels on the floor. Keep all four corners of the feet evenly anchored. With shins back, knees as wide as feet, upper thighbones in, begin folding at the knees; try to bring the thighs parallel to the floor. Lift the sitting bones to support you. Holding, lift the front hipbones from the thighs, body up as much as possible, as if sitting in a chair. Keep the chin parallel, gaze forwards, breath steady. Hold for 10 seconds; come to standing slowly.

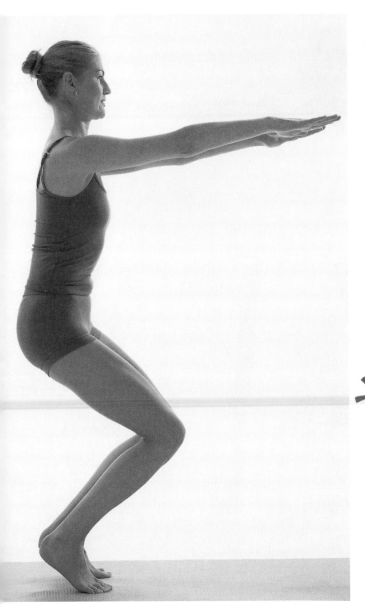

2 Lower the body

Keeping your toes relaxed and flat to the floor, shift your weight forwards and begin to lift your heels directly behind your ankles as high as you can. Now bend at the knees and lower your body as if sliding down a wall. Ideally, ears, shoulders, hips, and ankles look in line from the side. Come down 20-25 cm (8-10 inches): keep the front of your torso open and back to remain upright and aligned. As you hold your torso steady, keep lifting your heels, trying to bring your feet perpendicular to the floor. Again, keep your chin parallel to the floor, gaze forwards, breath smooth and steady. Hold for 10 seconds before slowly coming back to standing.

Hot tips Knees veer in or out of centre? Go back to the setting-up instructions to check your alignment and joint movement. When feet aren't evenly grounded and the ankle joints are not stabilised, weight rolls to the inside or outside of the feet. As your flexibility and strength balance out from hips to toes, you'll find it easier to hold everything in place.

3 Touch knees

Lift your heels and bend your knees slightly keeping your body upright. Turn your legs inward, bringing your knees to touch, heels and sitting bones out. Keep your knees glued together. Again, as if sliding down a wall, lower your hips, letting your knees come down and forwards, and trying to descend until your thighs are parallel with the floor. Keep your chin parallel to the floor, your gaze forwards, your breath smooth and steady. Hold for 10 seconds.

Hot tips Torso leaning forwards? This throws off your centre of gravity. Keep your side-view alignment the same as in step 2: ears, shoulders, hips and ankles all visibly in line.

COMING OUT Ascend slowly in the same way that you went down. Bring your feet back together and take your arms down to your sides.

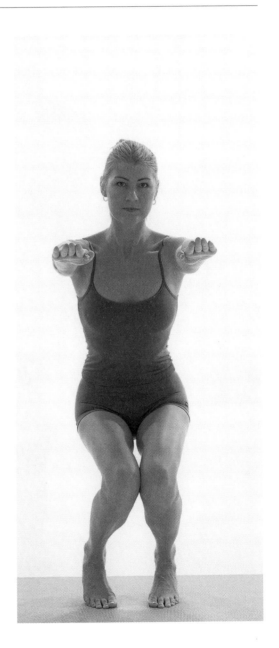

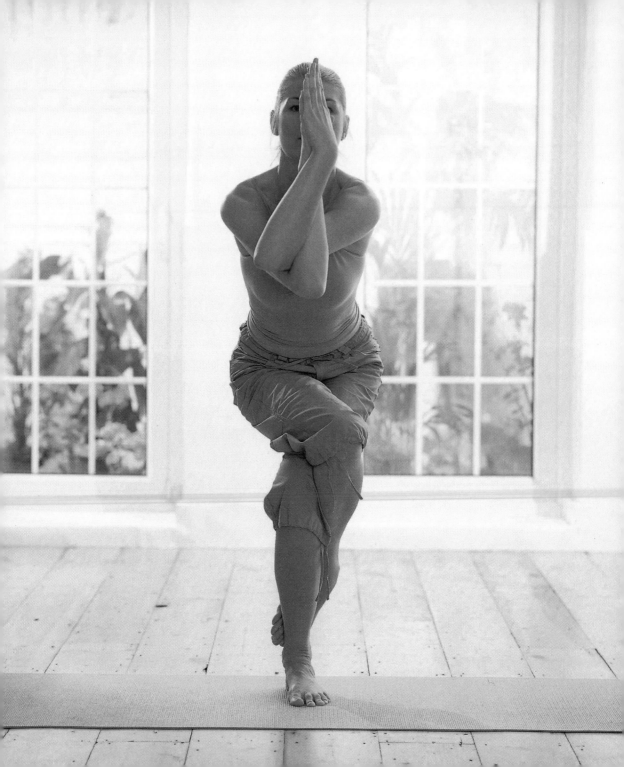

EAGLE POSE

GARUDASANA

This is the last pose in the warm-up phase of the standing series, named for *garuda,* the eagle. The extremities undergo a twisted-rope type maneuver as you balance in a seated position. The compression and release action of this pose stimulates the 12 major joints in the body–the ankles, knees, hips, shoulders, elbows and wrists–as well as the pelvic organs. It is also the first pose in which you start to explore balancing on one leg. After finishing this pose you are invited to take a quick water break before starting to work on the balancing standing postures.

STARTING POSITION: *standing at the centre of the mat facing the mirror.*

SETTING UP From Tadasana, inhale, raising your arms over your head while relaxing your shoulders away from your ears. Exhaling, gently swing your arms down and around the front of your body, crossing your right arm under your left at shoulder level. Bend your elbows and cross your wrists, palms facing upwards. Now bring your palms together in prayer position and cross thumbs.

Hot tips Overrounding and stretching the back when wrapping the arms? This closes the chest and abdominal cavity. Make sure you keep space at the front of the body to take the stretch to areas that are commonly neglected.

1 Arm position
Inhale width and length into the chest cavity, then, as you exhale, retain the space in your chest, draw your abdomen in and up, release your shoulders away from your ears and take your forearms and hands away from your face, directly above the elbows. Keep your head and neck in a neutral position.

Hot tips As you inhale, lengthen and widen the front of the body by opening the diamond points of the chest and pelvis (see page 23).

2 Fold forwards
Inhale again, maintaining the upper body setup. Exhaling, fold forwards from the hips, torso parallel to the floor. Inhale space into tight areas, then exhale and fold at the knees, taking the thighs parallel to the floor while keeping your chest open, spine neutral. Inhaling, rotate your pelvis away from your thighs to bring the torso up. Exhale and stabilise as you lift the right heel, toes on the floor, shifting weight off the right leg. Counterbalance the right hip off the left shoulder.

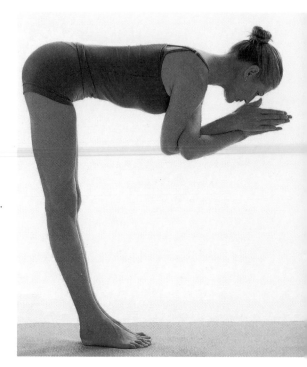

3 Leg position

Inhale and take your right thigh above your left thigh, allowing the right foot to hang below the right knee. Exhale and cross the legs, making an 'X' with your thighs, then compress the thighs into each other in a seated position. Inhale, drawing your right knee back to move the hip back, and exhale, leveling the hips and squaring up your torso. Working with the breath, bring your lower legs towards each other and reach the right foot around the left calf, hooking your big toe around the inner part of your left ankle. Continue working to close any gaps in your intertwined extremities while remaining seated upright with chest and abdomen open. Hold for 10 seconds.

COMING OUT At the end of an exhalation, slowly release your twisted arms and legs and, as you begin inhaling, stand up, bringing your arms overhead and exhaling them down and around to repeat the pose on the other side. This time, cross your left arm beneath your right arm, your left leg over your right leg. After holding on this side, exit the pose and immediately reenter on the right side to start a second set on both sides. Once you have released the left side for the second time, return to Tadasana, practicing stillness for two breaths.

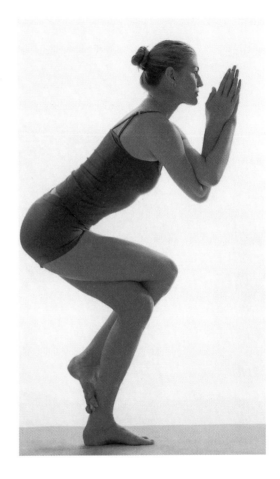

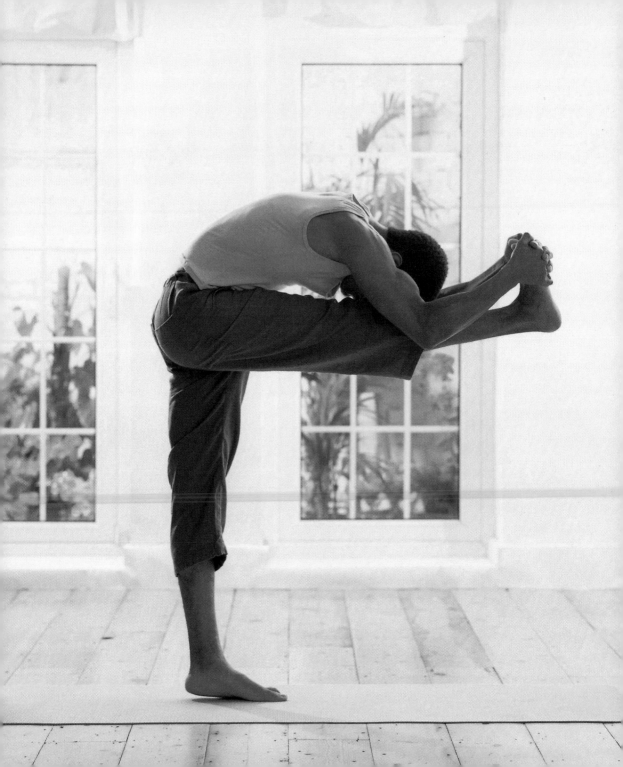

STANDING HEAD-TO-KNEE POSE

DANDAYAMANA-
JANUSHIRASANA

The following three standing poses introduce balancing on one leg–*danda* means a stick or staff. In all three, let your primary focus in the beginning be on keeping your standing leg straight and stable while you progress through the movements. Imagine you have no knee, your leg resembling a post from heel to hip. This first pose is a forward bend. Your long-term goal is to be able to stand on one leg and extend the other leg parallel to the floor with foot flexed and fingers interlaced behind it, elbows dropped below the calf and spine rounded over the extended leg, forehead touching the knee. This sounds like a phenomenal feat, and the finished pose is very impressive. However, your first goal is to develop increment by increment, and to strike a balance between strength and flexibility. It is more important to perfect the stages of development than to achieve the big picture.

STARTING POSITION: *standing at the centre of the mat facing the mirror.*

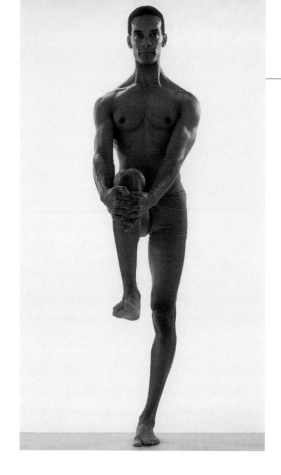

forwards, thigh back, lower leg in, upper leg out. These opposing actions stabilise the knee joint and keep it from bending. As you do this, pick up the right thigh to parallel. Keep your standing leg stable and torso square as you move the right leg.

1 Leg extension

Once you have established steadiness, pivot forwards from the hips, keeping your torso extended over your right thigh until your thigh is parallel with the floor. Keep your abdomen in and upper body up to prevent your centre of gravity from shifting forwards. Place your interlaced hands beneath the arch of your right foot and immediately kick your heel forwards, in line with the hip. Allow your arms to extend fully. Keep your chest open and up, away from the extended leg. Work on this stage until you can fully extend your right leg with foot flexed. Level your hips and square up your body.

Hot tips Rounding your spine over the extended leg? Extending the heel above or below the hip joint? Torso not staying square? Don't rush ahead without acknowledging the details: you won't develop the foundations necessary for support, and without support you can't adequately release inflexibility. The resistance between strength and flexibility simply exhausts your energy.

SETTING UP Standing with feet parallel, hip-width apart, lift your right heel and lightly rest the ball of your foot directly under your right hip, knee softly bent. Level out your hip line and square your shoulders. Aim to keep the diamond points of the chest and pelvis open wide (see page 23). Keep your shoulders relaxed, ears over your shoulders, chin parallel and eyes focused straight ahead. Begin to stabilise your left leg. Keeping ankle, knee and hip aligned, direct your muscular energy as follows: calf

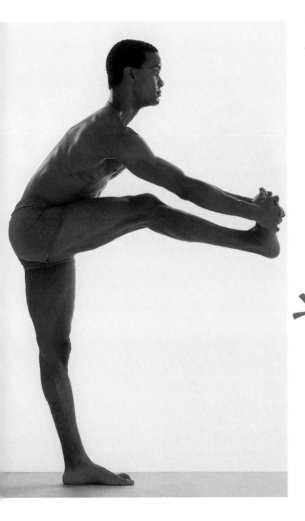

2 Lower the torso

Slowly fold in at the elbows, lowering your torso over the extended leg until your elbows are just below your calf. Once again, adjust any misalignment, then very slowly tuck your chin into your throat, pull back through your lower abdomen and, lifting up from the centre, place your forehead on your knee, as shown on page 60. Hold and breathe, aware that this pose is one minute long from beginning to end. As you develop the strength and flexibility required for steady movement, you will gain time to fine-tune this stage.

Hot tips Challenge yourself without making too many compromises, and whenever you lose your stability, back up, regain what you lost, and begin again to work with your breath to progress steadily through the process. When using the breath, inhale slowly, drawing in strength and space to areas that need them. As you exhale, stabilise and release into needy areas.

COMING OUT Release the pose with the same awareness you came into it, and return to Tadasana. Take a breath and begin setting up to work on the left side. After finishing this side, take two full breaths in Tadasana and begin a second set. This is only 30 seconds long: muscle memory allows the body to progress a little quicker to the stage you achieved in the first set.

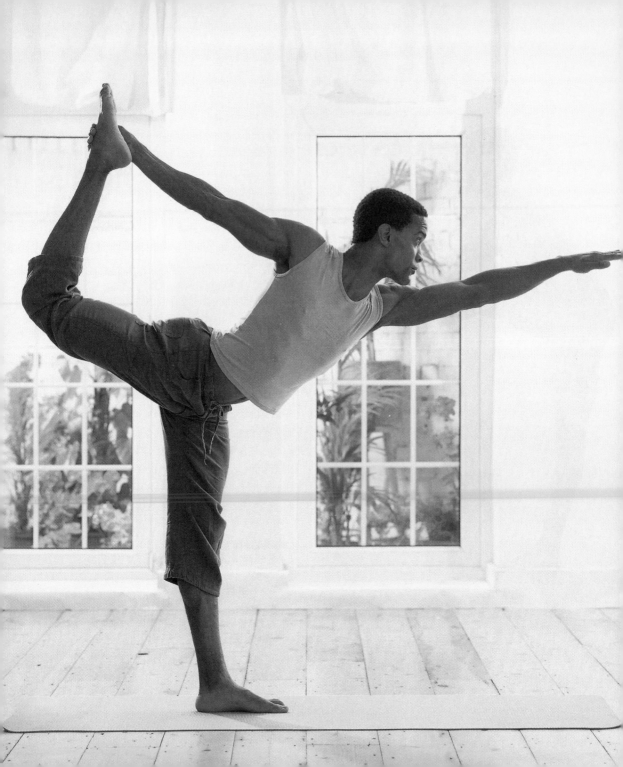

STANDING BOW PULLING POSE

DANDAYAMANA-DHANURASANA

The next challenge in your pursuit of standing-strength and balance is a backward bend-*dhanura* refers to the archer's bow that your spine begins to resemble in the ideal pose. Work towards this ultimate goal by standing and balancing on one leg while holding the opposite foot behind you, arching and then twisting the upper back while kicking your leg up to a standing split. As in the previous pose, progress is best developed by breaking down the posture into stages: only by doing this will you be able to work out and eventually resolve your unique personal combination of imbalances.

STARTING POSITION: *standing at the centre of the mat facing the mirror.*

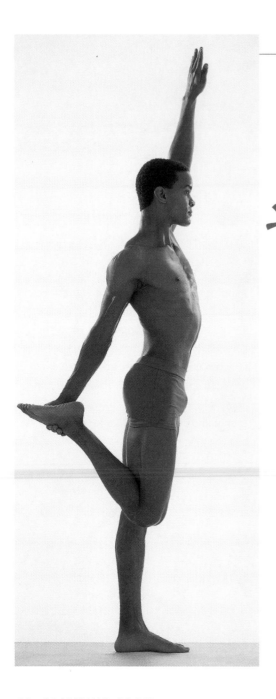

SETTING UP From Tadasana, release your bodyweight from your right leg while establishing the foundation in your left leg, then square up and level the torso just as you did when setting up the previous pose (see page 62).

Hot tips When you grab your foot, ensure that your shoulder does not rotate in towards your chest, closing it. Make sure, too, not to grab the outside of the foot, fry not to lift the shoulder and overextend the side of the body when holding the arm overhead. Progress to the next stage only when you feel happy with step 1.

Bend the leg

Rotate your right arm so the palm and inner elbow face out. Without tilting your pelvis forwards, extend your right leg behind, press the ball of the foot into the floor and straighten your leg (to pre-stretch the thigh and groin). Now draw your right heel to your buttock, pull your arm behind you without changing position, and cradle the arch side of your foot in your palm (thumb towards the toes, inner elbow facing out). Keep your hip-bones up, tailbone down as you bring your thighs together, knees in line. Take your left arm back and circle it overhead, palm forwards. Realign yourself, squaring your torso (equalise the length between underarm and hip on both sides, shoulders down and level, hips level) and stabilising your standing leg.

2 Pivot forwards

Slowly pivot from the hips, bringing your torso parallel to the floor. Kick your right heel away from your buttock as you begin to arch the upper back. Let the torso hang as you kick away just enough to keep yourself from falling forwards. Keeping the left leg stable, left shoulder in line with the hip, relax your right hip down until even with the left hip. Release your left shoulder from your ear while lengthening your right side from hip to underarm to square the body.

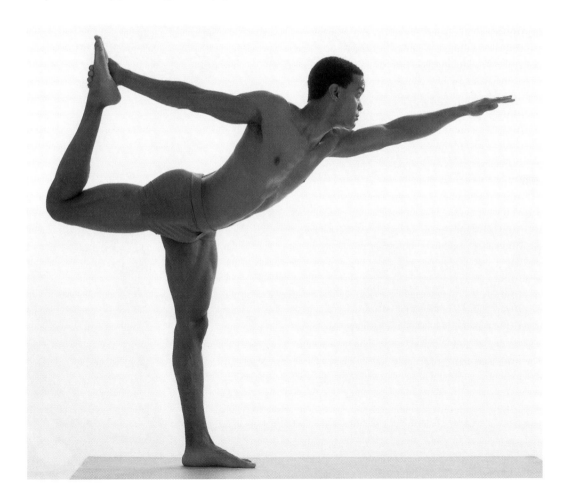

WORKING THE POSE Work on developing evenness in both sides of the body, continuing to open the chest by bending the upper back, and continuing to stretch the right groin by kicking the leg back into your hand and straight up. Keep your hips stabilised on top of your standing leg, and stretch your rib cage away from your hips. Bend your upper back backward, let your extended leg pull your arm back to open the chest and feel your extended arm lengthen and pull back into the shoulder, keeping both shoulders in line. Make sure your right and left joints stay aligned. Maintain enough tension between the kick back into your hand and the body movement down (chest up) to prevent yourself from falling forwards.

Hot tips Joints of the standing leg not aligned? Move your thigh forwards, bringing hip and ankle joints in line, then straighten the leg. If your hips are not level, draw the standing leg in and up, then relax your opposite hip down, keeping the torso square. If the shoulder of your front arm moves forwards, causing the body to shift off centre, draw the arm back to move the shoulder back, and stretch into the opposite armpit to equalise the length of your sides, then align yourself to find your centre. Don't move to the next stage until you feel confident here.

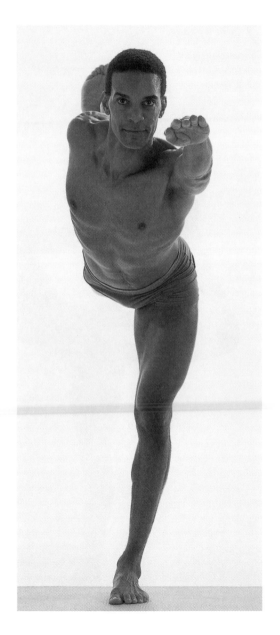

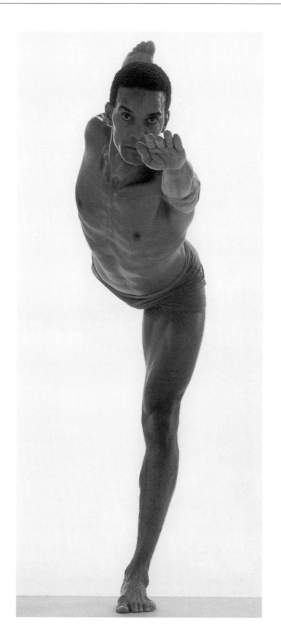

3 Spinal twist

Maintaining the integrity of the pose you achieved in step 1, begin to twist the chest while continuing to kick up into the standing splits. Your arms, shoulders and extended leg eventually align in the centre. Let your hand slide to the ankle as your leg goes up. The legs rotate inward as they split. Practice for 1 minute on the first set.

WORKING THE POSE Use your breath to breathe your way to your edges and begin to play at the edge as you continue to maintain integrity and work on your weaknesses. Once you have reached this stage, you might like to start the pose with feet slightly pigeon-toed and legs slightly rotated.

COMING OUT Exit the pose with awareness, reversing the steps you used to enter the pose, and return to Tadasana. Work on the left side, then repeat on both sides, this time holding for 30 seconds.

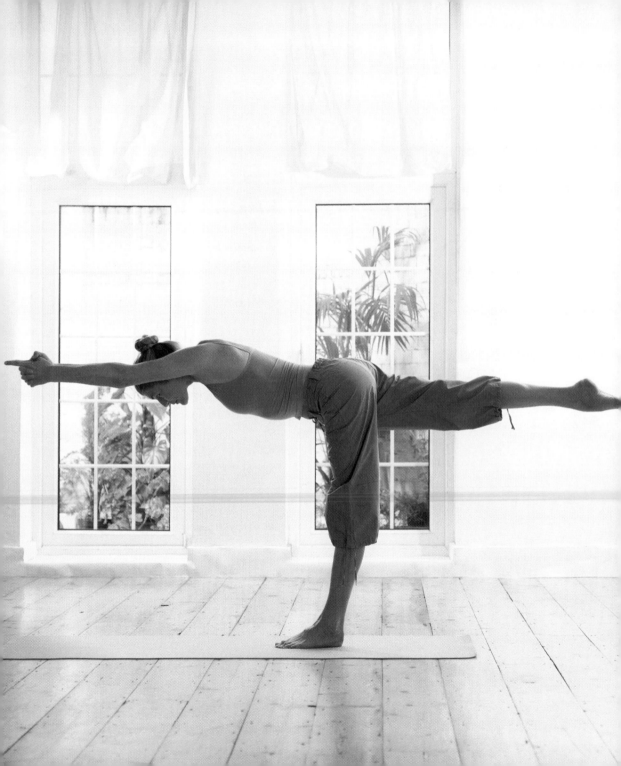

BALANCING STICK

TULADANDASANA

Often referred to as putting the body into a 'T' formation, this is the final standing strength-building pose. You try to hold the body in a stable neutral position parallel with the floor while balancing on one leg. There is nothing to kick or pull against in this balancing position; it is all about stabilisation. Although the pose is held for only 10 seconds, it has a noticeable effect on the heart. When you bring the arms overhead and then take the body and extended leg parallel to the floor, there is a sudden increase in the amount of blood returning to the heart, causing it to contract harder in order to pump blood back out to the body. The heart is a muscle and this action strengthens it–in this posture you exercise your heart while developing grace.

STARTING POSITION: *standing at the back of the mat facing the mirror.*

SETTING UP Make sure you have enough room in front to step forwards and bend forwards with arms overhead. From Tadasana, take your arms overhead on an inhalation and interlace your fingers, releasing your index fingers like a steeple. Exhale and draw your forearms together, straightening your elbows and wrists. Release your arms down into the shoulder sockets, and relax your shoulders away from your ears (see setting up for Half-Moon Pose with Hands-to-Feet Pose, page 46).

Hot tips Move back your front thighs, back ribs, back of the head and arms to align the side-view centre of your body. Feel your front-view centre aligned through your inner legs, pubis, navel, sternum, centre of the chin, nose and inner wrists through your palms.

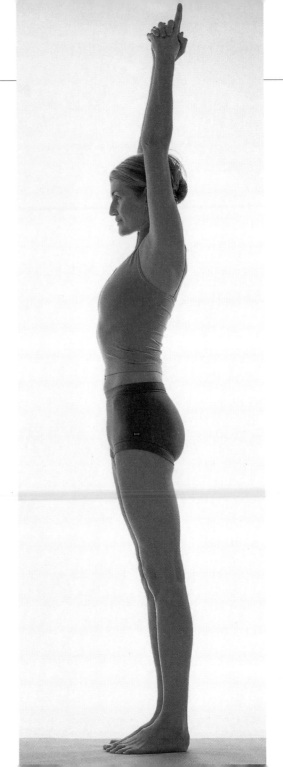

1 Lift the leg

Inhale and step forwards with your right foot, coming to stand with all the leg joints aligned. Exhale, tilting your pelvis forwards and aligning head and body with your left leg. Inhale, draw energy into the standing leg, and rotate the other leg inward while pressing through the width of the ball of the foot. Exhale and stabilise. Inhale, opening the front of the body to square the torso, and lift your extended leg slightly up from the floor while stabilising the entire body. As you exhale, pivot forwards with control from the hips, maintaining joint alignment and stability, to bring your body and extended leg parallel with the floor, as shown on page 70. Keep your chest down and arms up, head between the arms. At the same time rotate the extended leg inward as you hold it level with the hip. Work at your edge (see page 17) for 10 seconds. As you inhale, reach down through the supporting foot and draw energy up to the hip for support. As you exhale, stretch across to the opposite hip and level the hips while stretching the ribs away.

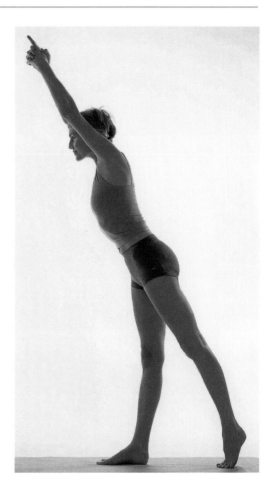

Hot tips Don't let the chest collapse and spine round forwards: this looks more like an umbrella than a 'T.' Pivot in a straight line from the hip joint. Be aware of side-bending when pivoting forwards: pay attention to aligning your right and left sides and move slowly, backing up and making corrections before continuing.

COMING OUT On an inhalation, pivot back up until your extended leg touches the ground. Step back with your standing leg and bring your arms down to your sides. Take two full breaths and then begin to work on the left side. Repeat a second set on both sides.

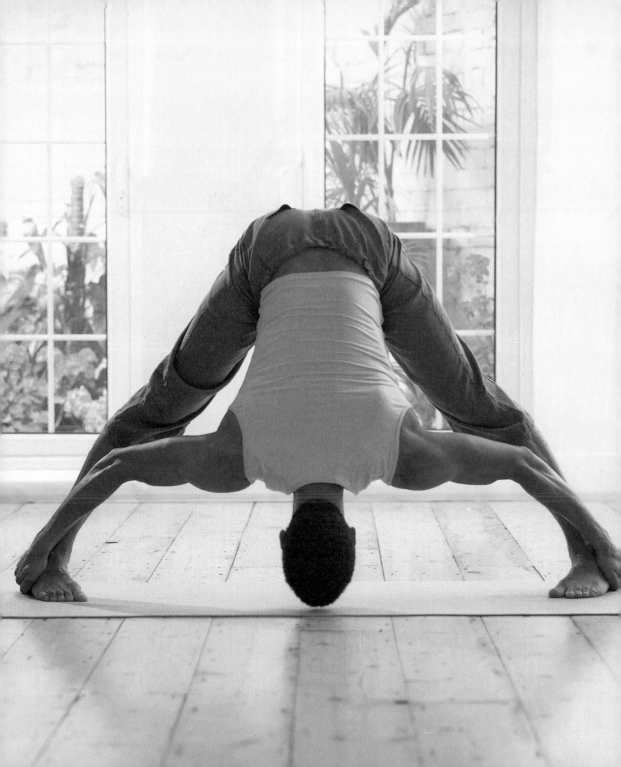

STANDING SEPARATE LEG STRETCHING POSE

DANDAYAMANA-BIBHAKTAPADA-PASCHIMOTTHANASANA

The next three standing poses are practiced with legs separated, and work the inner thighs, outer thighs and hips. In the first pose, your long-term goal is to be able to stand with straight legs separated 94-122 cm (3-4 feet) apart, folding forwards from the hips with your spine in a neutral position to place your forehead on the floor between your feet. To maximise your opportunity to develop the necessary flexibility in the legs, hips and lower back, keep your shoulders and chest squared up with your hips, and allow the forwards pelvic rotation to be the movement that takes you to your edge.

STARTING POSITION: *move the mat to give a side-on view in the mirror; stand at the left end of the mat.*

SETTING UP Standing in Tadasana, inhale and take your arms overhead. Exhaling, step your right leg as far to the right as you comfortably can while bringing your arms down in line with your shoulders. Place your feet parallel, heels in line, and align your joints all the way up, ears over shoulders, chin neutral.

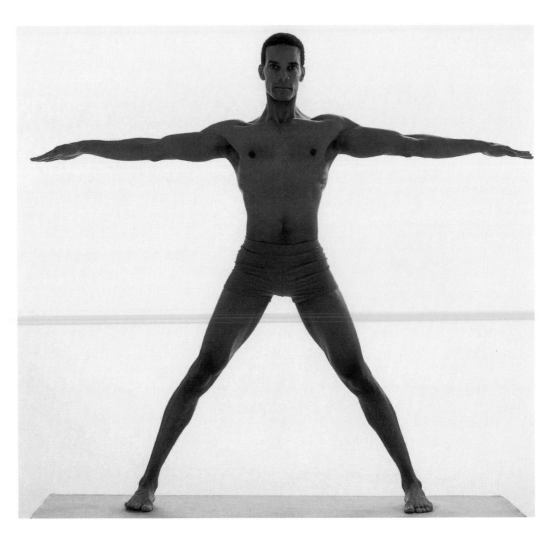

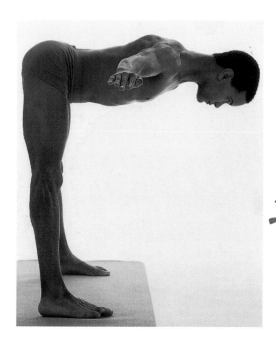

Fold forwards

Exhale and begin folding forwards from the hips (a pelvic rotation). Work with your breath and maintain the alignment in the upper and lower body. Inhale, drawing strength and space into the appropriate opposing areas. Exhale and stabilise, releasing any gripping and relaxing deeper into the pose.

Hot tips Hips behind your heels, legs angling back? You won't achieve a full calf stretch. To remedy this, bring your legs forwards until your hips are directly above your ankles. Take your calves forwards, thighs back until the knees are centred between the hip and ankle joints. If the hip and ankle joints are aligned but your knee pushes back, soften behind the knee and centre it with the ankle and hip by taking your calf forwards and thigh back. This stabilises the knee in the centre of these joints. Watch out also when the chest collapses and the upper spine rises above the curvature of the lower spine, which overstretches the upper spine. Work on opening the chest and pelvic diamonds (see page 23).

Stabilise

Inhaling, stabilise the legs (draw down through your feet and up through your legs, keeping both sides of the feet on the floor and outer ankles pulled in; bring the energy in the lower legs in and forwards, the upper legs apart and back, joints stacked in a perpendicular line). Exhale and release any gripping without losing stability. Inhaling, stabilise the spine in a neutral position (create space in the front of the pelvis and chest, lift your pelvic floor and relax the buttocks and shoulders). Inhale and acknowledge the stability in both areas.

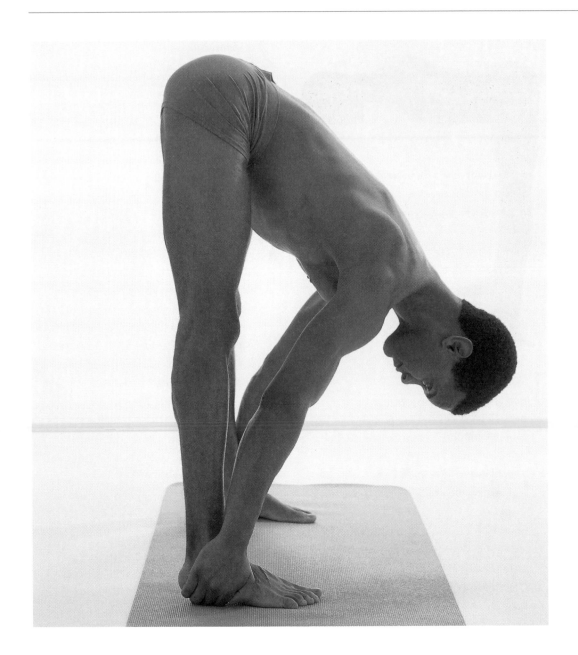

3 Introduce the arms

Once your torso has rotated around your legs enough, reach back with your arms and grab your calves, ankles, or, depending on your flexibility, cup your hands beneath your heels. Apply a gentle pulling action to the stretch. Make sure your chest stays open and squared with the hips, your spine remains neutral. Inhale, drawing strength and space into the appropriate opposing areas. Exhale, stabilising and relaxing any gripping and, as you release deeper into the pose, fold into the elbows. Draw through your elbow fold away from the centre (this really opens the chest and stabilises the upper spine as you fold in deeper at the groin crease). Lift up through the crease and move your body closer to your legs. Hold for 20 seconds.

WORKING THE POSE Once you can maintain a neutral spine and straight legs while folding your body into your legs, bring your chin away from your throat without crunching the back of the neck so the forehead rather than crown of the head sits between your feet.

COMING OUT Stabilise, then reverse the moves that took you into the pose. Inhaling, come up with a neutral spine and stable, strong legs. Exhaling, step your right leg to the left, arms back to your sides in Tadasana for two breaths. Repeat a second set.

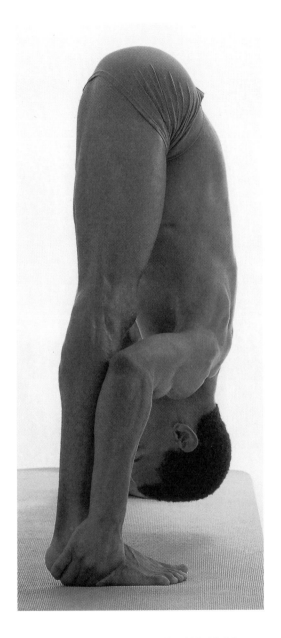

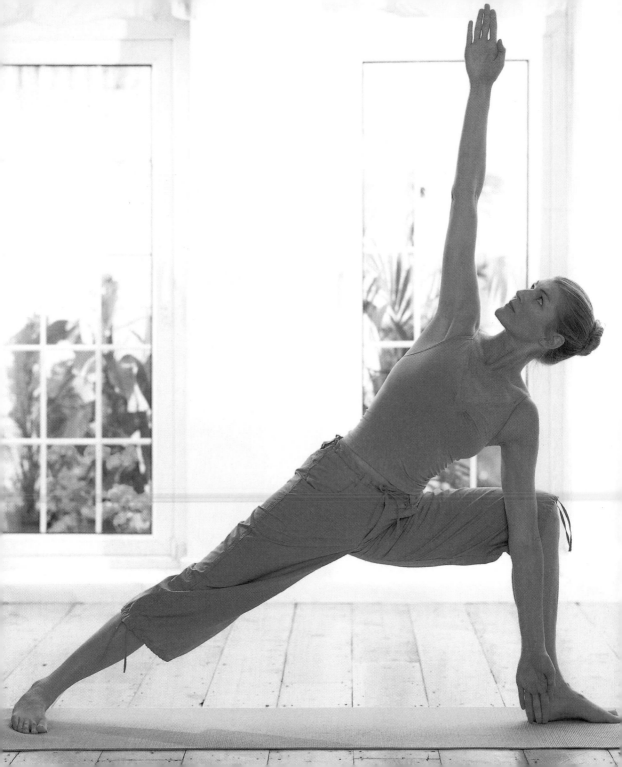

TRIANGLE POSE

TRIKONASANA

A blend of several standing postures, known in traditional hatha yoga as the Extended Triangle (Utthita Trikonasana), Warrior II (*Virabhadrasana* II), and Extended Side Angle poses (Utthita Parsvakonasana), this position, with its external rotation of the legs and forwards rotation of the pelvis, creates a stretch in the inner thighs as the hips open up. There are many opposing factors to bear in mind while you work, and it really puts your overall strength and hip flexibility to the test. Setting up the foundations well will equip you to overcome this pose's multiple obstacles, and will allow you to enjoy stretching into the angles, leaving you feeling as powerful as a warrior.

STARTING POSITION: *turn the mat lengthwise to the mirror so you see the front-view alignment; start at the left end of the mat facing the mirror.*

SETTING UP From Tadasana, inhale and bring your arms overhead. Exhale and step your right foot as far to the right as you can while bringing your arms down to shoulder-level, palms facing down. Turn your palms up, inhale, expand the width of your chest, and rotate your inner elbows up. Exhale and turn your palms down. Turn your right foot to a 12 o'clock position, your left foot to 10 o'clock. Inhaling, lift the inner part of your front knee and thigh, and rotate this leg outward. Exhale and draw your upper leg bone in and up under the hip, providing support for the body. Stretch the outer edge of your left foot into the floor while drawing the outer ankle in; stabilise the leg with the kneecap lifted.

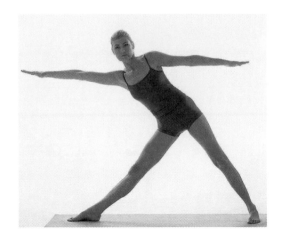

1 Fold to the side

Keeping the inner knee of your front leg lifted and the thigh spiraling up under the hip, inhale and soften into the groin crease while bringing your right arm straight up over the shoulder, palm facing forwards. Exhale and fold to the side, drawing in at the groin while reaching upwards through your right arm to create a sideways 'V' formation (>) with your right arm and torso and right leg. Align the left side of your torso with your left leg. Inhale while re-establishing your foundations, and soften into the right groin and back of the knee.

Exhaling, continue to draw into the fold of the groin and knee, sending the knee towards the heel and making the thigh parallel. The knee must never go beyond the ankle. If flexibility permits, slide your left heel back, deepening the angle formed at the groin.

Hot tips Front leg rotates internally with the knee in front of the ankle and hip? Back up and re-establish your foundations: lift your inner knee and thigh, and rotate the leg outward. Then draw the upper leg bone in and up beneath the hip for support. Stretch the outer edge of your left foot into the floor while drawing the outer ankle in, and stabilise the leg, kneecap lifted. If the toes of your back foot lift from the floor, keep the ball of that foot stretched wide into the floor; this also boosts stabilisation.

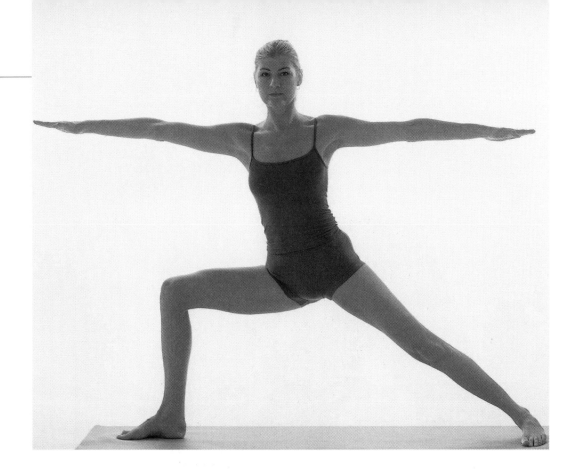

2 Complete the triangle

Keeping the right shoulder up, swing the right arm like a pendulum to hang straight down. At the same time, bring your left arm up in a perpendicular line with shoulders and arms. Keep your right side over the thigh; firm your arms, right arm pressing back against the leg. Drop your head to align neck and spine. Turn the head left to align chin and shoulder; look at the thumb, as on page 80. Hold for 10 seconds: inhale into foundations and folds; exhale, stabilise; rotate torso and left leg away.

COMING OUT Inhaling, turn the head back to centre, lift your right arm and drop your left arm to bring your arms back to parallel while you straighten your right leg. Exhale, turn your left foot to a 12 'clock position, your right foot to 2 o'clock, and continue setting up to work on the left side. When finished on the left, turn the feet parallel and inhale the arms overhead. Exhale, bringing your right leg to meet the left and taking your arms to your sides. Take two breaths, before beginning a second set on both sides.

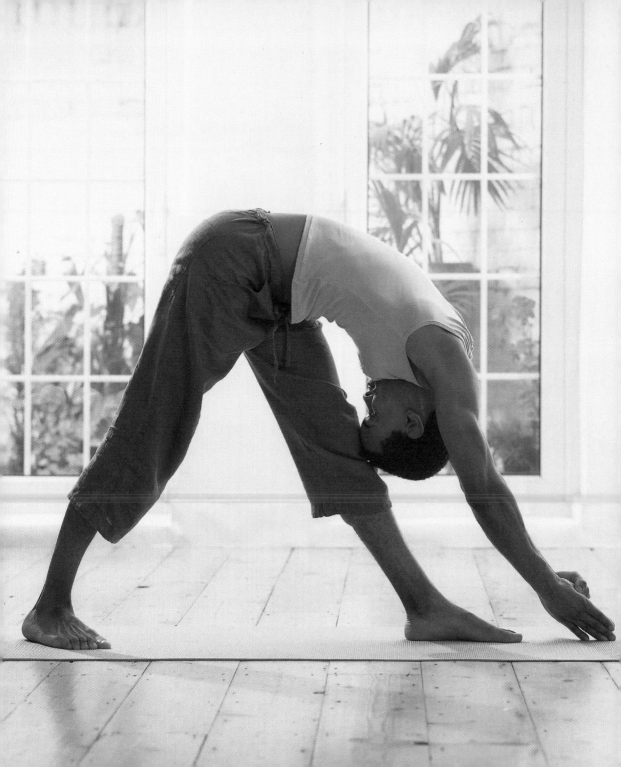

STANDING SEPARATE LEG HEAD-TO-KNEE POSE

DANDAYAMANA-BIBHAKTAPADA-JANUSHIRSASANA

This pose closes the hips and simultaneously lengthens the spine as you round your back and tuck your forehead above your knee (*sirsa* means head and *janu* knee). The internal rotation of the legs and forwards rotation of the pelvis provide a stretch to the sides of the thighs and hips. To maximise the stretching of the posterior spine, make sure you first achieve a stretch in areas where the spine arches–the back of the neck and lower back. Then continue rounding to create a more even stretch along the entire length of the spine. This posture gives a deep contraction and compression to the throat and abdomen, which stimulates the organs and glands, especially the thyroid gland, whose hormonal secretions are responsible for regulating many of the body's physiological functions.

STARTING POSITION: *turn the mat back so that the top of the mat faces the mirror; stand at the left end of the mat, right side towards the mirror.*

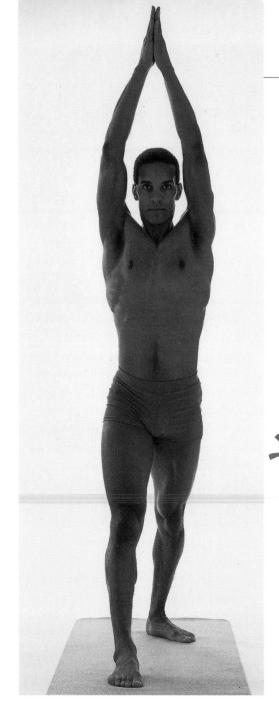

SETTING UP From Tadasana, inhale, bringing your arms overhead and placing your palms together with thumbs crossed. Exhaling, step your right leg approximately 91 cm (3 feet) to the right. Pivoting on the balls of the feet, turn right to face the front of the mat and place your front foot parallel with the edge of the mat, leg straight. Turn your hips a few more times to the right as you bring your back heel around behind your left toes, stretching the ball of the foot into the floor while straightening your leg. Square up your torso towards the mirror. Without turning your left hip away, place your back heel down in line with your front heel, bending your front knee if necessary (in a lunge position).

Hot tips Legs not stable? Bend your front knee into a lunge, plant your foot firmly down and stabilise the leg. Then straighten your back leg as you press through the ball of the foot to begin stretching the leg. Slowly stretch your heel to the ground.

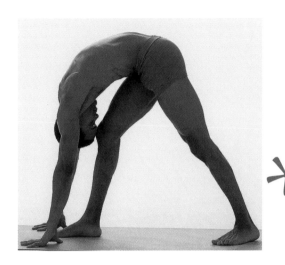

WORKING THE POSE Continue to stretch your backside by evenly holding open the inner circle you have formed in connecting head to knee as you gently push your knee back with your head to straighten the front leg. Aim to take your hands in front of the foot, palms together in prayer position (as on page 84).

Hot tips Hips and/or shoulders not square? Veer to the side when bending forwards? Change your foot position to give better alignment and stability. Also pay close attention when moving forwards and curling in that your right and left sides are aligned.
When the chin is drawn back and up, the throat feels choked. Compressing and contracting the abdomen and chest makes it even more difficult to breathe. To be effective in the posture, surrender to the situation by remaining calm. Very slowly and gently bring the breath in as deeply as possible to areas of restriction, then slowly exhale, releasing deeper into the pose.

1 Round forwards

Inhaling, internally rotate your legs and, back heel down, exhale and pivot the hips forwards slightly, increasing the stretch to the back of the leg to a comfortable edge while stretching the buttocks. Inhale, draw chin to throat, then exhale, lifting into the throat while drawing into the groin crease. Inhale space into the back of the neck and pelvis, tuck the chin towards the base of the throat to hold the cervical stretch; at the same time, press the lower abdomen into the pelvis to hold the lumbar stretch. Exhale, drawing the torso back into the spine as you contract the abdomen and chest. Round forwards evenly, right eyebrow above knee, nose aligned with inner thigh, hands either side of the front foot.

COMING OUT Inhale and untuck your chin. Exhaling, stretch forwards and stabilise your spine and legs. Inhale and come up. As you exhale, pivot on the balls of the feet all the way to the left, facing the back of the mat. Repeat the pose. After coming up on an inhalation, exhale and pivot halfway to the right. Inhale, taking your arms overhead, and step your right leg to the left. Exhale your arms back to your sides. Take two full breaths before beginning a second set on both sides.

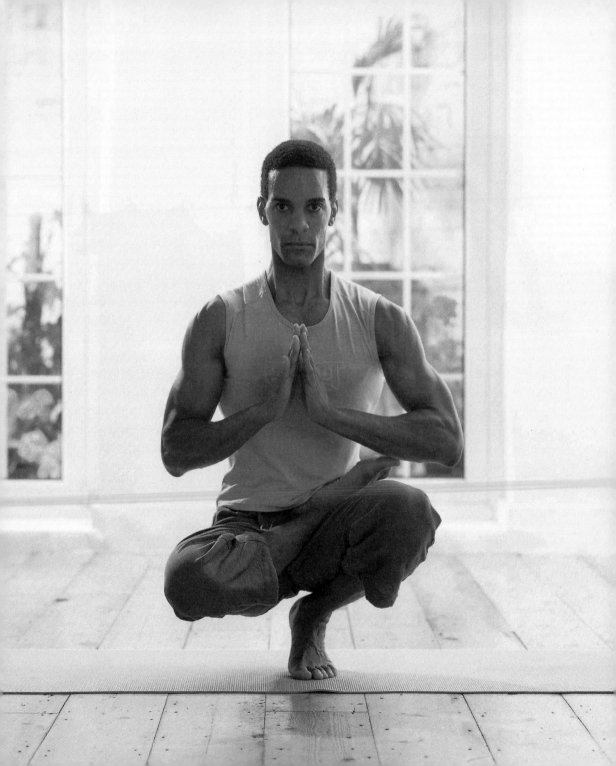

STABILISING

TREE POSE AND TOE STAND POSE

TADASANA VRKASANA–
PADANGUSTASANA

The stability of the mountain and tree (*tada* and *vrksa* in Sanskrit) are recalled in the final standing poses that challenge you to stand upright, stabilising and balancing on one leg while you work on opening the hips, stretching the inside of the opposite leg into a half-lotus position (Tree Pose). The second set of this pose has an optional challenge–the Toe Stand. This is very hard on the knees if inflexibility is an issue for you, and is not recommended for students with any kind of knee injury, nor for beginners, who may not have the flexibility required to achieve this advanced level of control and steadiness.

STARTING POSITION: *standing in the centre of the mat, facing the mirror.*

SETTING UP From Tadasana, release your weight from your right leg and rest the ball of your right foot on the floor beneath your right hip. Inhale and begin to fine-tune your standing alignment while relaxing behind the knee and in the crease at the groin.

1 Fold the leg

Exhale, stabilise, and bring your right thigh up parallel to the floor. Inhale, open up across the front of the hips and move your right leg away from centre without allowing your hips to follow. Exhale and bring your right calf up to meet the back of your thigh. Inhale, stretching your toes evenly away from your ankle, keeping the outer part of the ankle drawn in. Exhaling, pivot slightly forwards from the hips, reach down through your legs with palms facing forwards, and grab the outside of your right ankle. Inhale and stretch your foot and knee back while drawing your sitting bone and ankle forwards to allow the hip and inner leg to open to their maximum extent. Exhale and bring your knee in towards the centre and back. Rest your right foot against the opposite thigh, eventually up in the crease of the groin, knees aligned. At the same time open up the front of your body, standing in balance as if in the basic standing pose for 10 seconds.

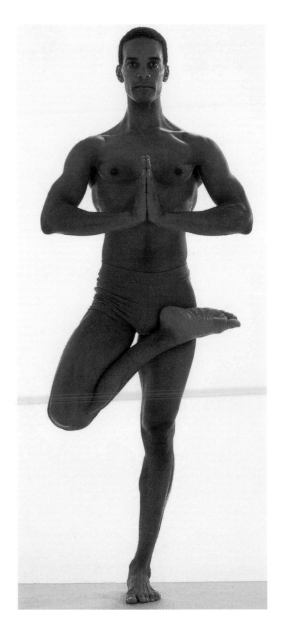

⁕ **Hot tips** Ankle sinks towards your thigh? Press the top of the foot towards the thigh and lift your ankle away, creating an opening along the entire length of the leg up to the hip.

Arching your back in order to stand upright? Instead, lift your folded knee, open your chest and pelvis, and stabilise before lowering the knee.

COMING OUT Stabilise, then lift your right leg, release the foot under the knee and set the foot back down beneath the hip. Centre yourself in Tadasana, then begin to work on your left side. After completing this side, take two breaths in Tadasana then set up for a second set on each side, starting on the right.

2 Optional Toe Stand (second set only)

To progress to the Toe Stand, at the end of step 1, fold forwards evenly from the hips and place your hands on the floor. Look at the floor approximately 122 cm (4 feet) ahead (do not move your eyes; keep the head in a neutral position with the spine) as you rise up on the ball of the foot of the standing leg, then sit down just above the heel. Lift your body as you come up on to fingertips, drop your right leg to the level of the left leg and draw them together. Draw in and up, bringing your body upright, lifting your hands into prayer position at chest level, as shown on page 88.

⁕ **Hot tips** You might like to try an intermediate position between steps 1 and 2 to help you towards the sitting toe stand. From the upright Tree Pose in step 1, fold forwards, place your hands to the floor and work with your breath to create the control you need to progress.

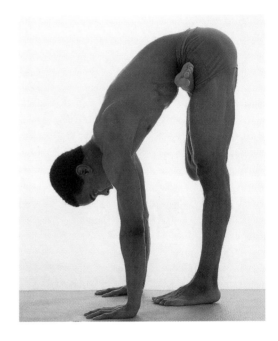

COMING OUT Place your hands back on the floor and raise your hips to straighten the standing leg. Stabilise; come up into upright Tree Pose. Release your folded leg, then repeat on the other leg. Stand still for two breaths. Lie back on the mat for two minutes.

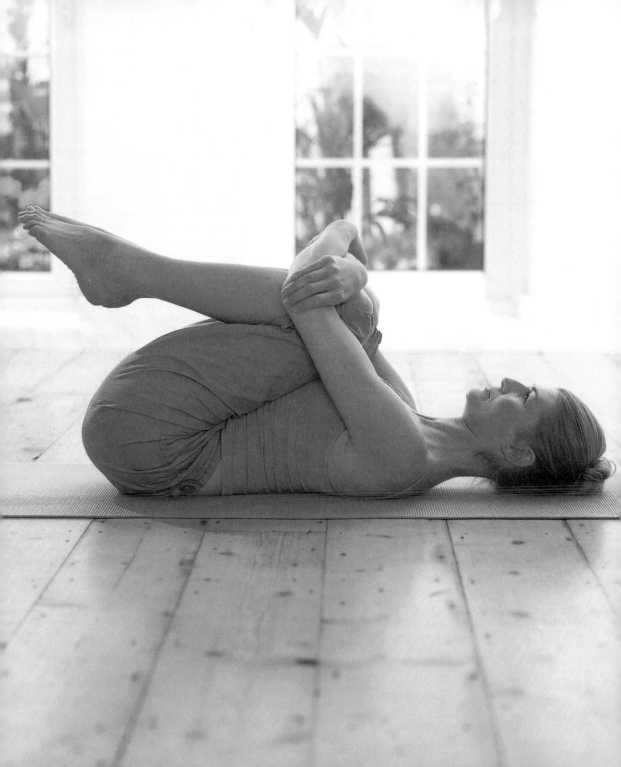

WIND-REMOVING POSE

PAVANAMUKTASANA

After a brief two-minute rest in Savasana (see page 36), the first of the floor postures compresses the lower abdomen, stimulating the peristaltic action of the colon and therefore removing trapped gas (in the Sanskrit, *pavana* refers to breath, in this case air, and *mukta* means free from). The pose provides much the same stretch as the first standing balance (Standing Head-to-Knee, pages 60-63). Understanding the resemblance between these poses allows you to work a similar stretch using a different approach, increasing your awareness of the complete picture. Here, you do not have to struggle with balancing on one leg and so are able to move your focus to the obstacles found when you maintain the foundation of an open, squared-up torso. In so doing, you develop the flexibility for safe forward bending. There are three parts to each set in the stretch.

STARTING POSITION: *top of the mat towards the mirror; lying on your back with your head at the top of the mat.*

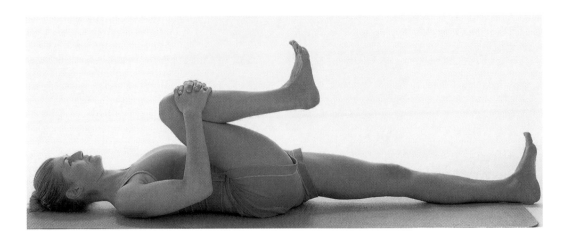

SETTING UP Lying on your back, extend your legs straight out from your hips with feet flexed, as if standing on the floor. Keeping your chest and pelvis open, ground down beneath your shoulder blades and hip bones to stabilise an open torso and prevent side bending.

1 Fold the right leg

Inhale space into the front of the body as you soften into the right side of the groin and knee-fold. Slide your right heel towards your right sitting bone while keeping the joints aligned and squared up. Flex your foot and toes, keep the outer ankle in and press through the ball of the foot to maximise the stretch and equalise the stretching of both the inner and outer parts of the leg.

Exhaling, stabilise your torso while lifting your right foot off the floor, and place your hands, fingers interlaced, below your knee-cap. Soften into the folds of the knee, groin and elbow as you fold your right leg into your body and bring your elbows to your sides. Work with your breath for 10 seconds as the compression stimulates the ascending colon. Release, reversing the folding action to extend the leg.

Hot tips Hip lifts towards the shoulder? Don't allow this to happen—it results in side bending and loss of foundation. Try anchoring your opposite shoulder down and back, then stretch diagonally into the lower part of the outer hip while bringing the leg in and up.

2 Fold the left leg

Reestablish your foundation: keeping your chest and pelvis open, ground down beneath your shoulder blades and hipbones to stabilise an open torso and prevent side bending. Repeat step 1 on the other side of the body, bringing your left leg in over your left side to compress and stimulate the descending colon.

Hot tips   Foot, lower leg and upper leg don't align when you fold one leg in? Keep the foundation in your body and move your foot away from centre as you pull the outer part of your ankle in, squaring the foot with the lower leg. Soften behind the knee and groin, the width of the joint, then bring your lower leg in and upper leg out, aligning the legs so they fold in evenly behind the knee. Continue folding the leg over your lower abdomen without losing your foundation. The inner ankle and lower leg lengthen, as do the outer hip and upper leg.

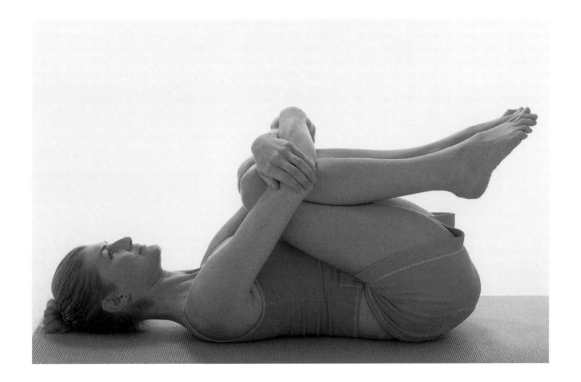

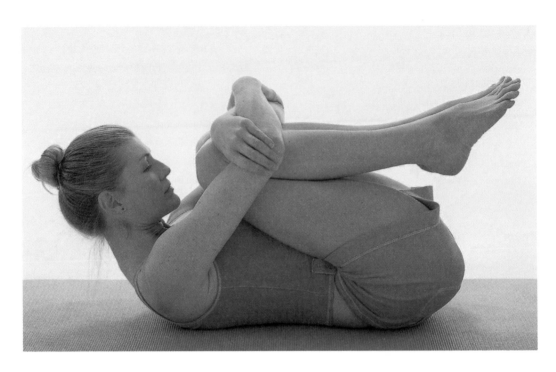

3 Bring both legs in

Reestablish your foundation and bring both heels towards your sitting bones. Inhale, opening the front of the body from the top of the shoulders to the groin creases. To increase your foundation points, stretch down into the groin creases while lifting your feet a few inches off the floor. Maintain this openness and, exhaling, bring your legs together and down over your lower abdomen. Inhale, and, lifting your spine into your thighs, rise up and wrap your arms around your folded legs, grabbing the opposite elbow if possible, as shown on page 95. If this is difficult, grasp the opposite forearm, wrist, or hand. Roll back, placing your upper back and head on the floor. Begin working with your breath to open the front of the body and allow the spine to move back in as the sides of the body begin to come to the floor. Ultimately, the back of the body rests evenly on the floor while you hold your folded legs against the lower part of your abdomen, a compression that stimulates the transverse colon. Work with your breath for 10 seconds.

Hot tips Don't close off the front of the body when lifting and wrapping the arms. Watch when pulling both legs in that your lower abdomen does not pull away from the thighs. This prevents the groin from exerting deep compression into the lower abdomen, and may overstretch segments of the lumbar (lower) spine.

COMING OUT Release your arms to your sides. Inhale, reestablish your initial foundation and lift your thighs away from your body, bringing your feet down to the floor. Exhale, slide, or baby-step your heels away from your sitting bones to straighten the legs. Relax for two breaths in Savasana (see pages 36–37) before beginning a second set.

WORKING THE POSE If you are strong enough to maintain the foundation when exiting the pose, keep your heels slightly off the floor and move them away until the legs straighten; then set your legs to the floor. This requires more abdominal strength to stabilise the pelvis.

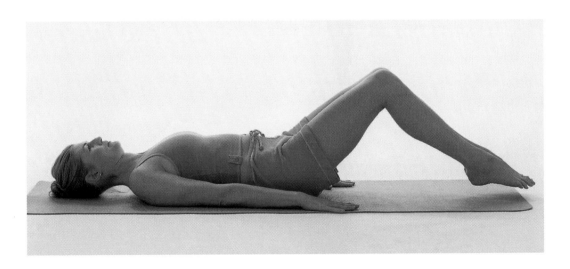

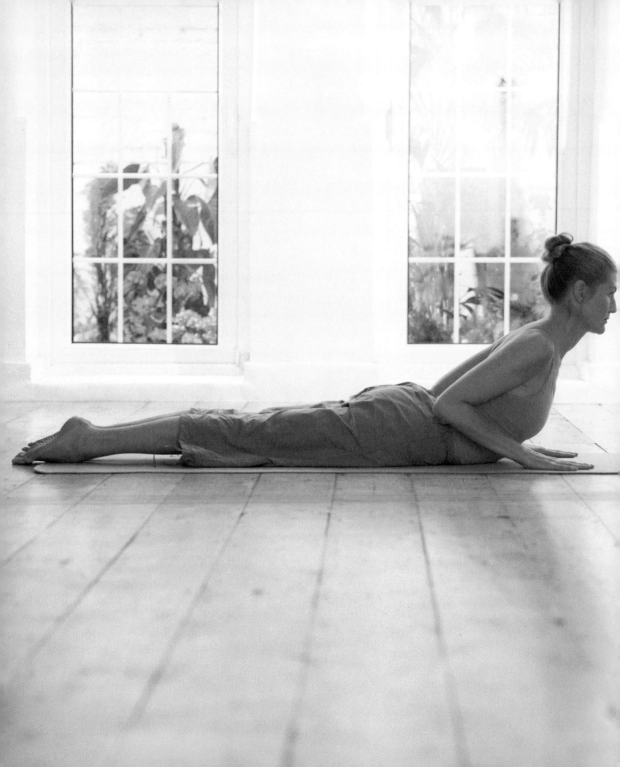

COBRA POSE

BHUJANGASANA

With this floor pose begins the spine-strengthening series of postures, which also prepare the body for backward bending. There are four postures: the first three isolate and strengthen a different segment of the spine, while the fourth works the entire spine. From the Sanskrit *bhujang,* meaning snake or serpent, the Cobra Pose focuses on strengthening the lower back. Additionally, it develops the back of the neck and thighs and opens the chest. These instructions are not for a full Cobra Pose, but a variation commonly referred to as Baby Cobra.

STARTING POSITION: *on hands and knees in the centre of the mat, facing the mirror.*

SETTING UP From the hands and knees position, with the tops of your feet at the back end of the mat, bring the inner sides of your feet, ankles, knees and thighs together. Place your hands forwards on the mat, chest-width apart, and begin to relax the back of the body forwards, bringing the thighs, pelvis, abdomen and chest (in that order) down on to the mat. As your chest comes down, stretch back through the crease of the elbows and slide your palms back so that your hands and fingers sit directly beneath your shoulders. Make sure your fingertips are in line with the top of the shoulders, little fingers with the outside edge, chest resting between your hands. Bring your head down, ears in line with your shoulders, nose lightly touching the mat, to establish a neutral spine before beginning the pose.

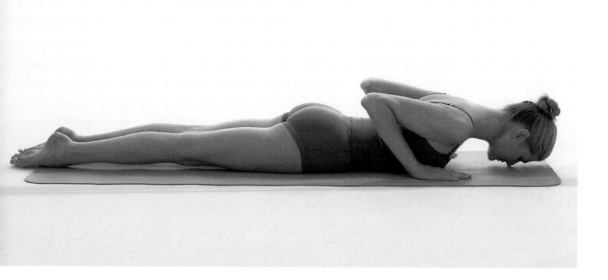

1 Establish a foundation

Keeping the top of the feet, front of the pelvis and abdomen on the floor, inhale, lifting your knees and navel up (engage the thighs and navel centre) while drawing your tailbone down towards the pubis. Do not allow your ribs to lift from the floor. Exhale, stabilising your foundation while relaxing your chest open.

Hot tips A sure sign of lack of foundation is the top of the feet and tailbone lifting from the floor, compressing the lower back. To remedy this, maintain contact with the floor from belly to toes while engaging the thighs and navel centre.

2 Lift the upper body

Inhale, lifting the upper body (lower rib to top of head) away from the floor. Do not push away using your hands. Exhale and arch the upper back as you draw back through the elbow crease, shoulders, throat and face. Move the upper part of the spine forwards, stretching open across the chest. Keep your hands free from weight, shoulders down away from your ears, and chin in a neutral position, as shown on page 100. Work with your breath to create a solid foundation while opening the chest. Find your edge, hold and breathe.

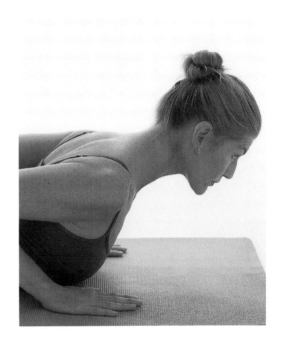

Hot tips Pressing your hands into the floor? Lifting your belly with your chest? Compressing the lumbar spine by arching? Lower your upper body and reestablish your foundation. Do not lift higher than the bottom of your ribs, nor any higher than you have the strength to hold. Draw back through the elbow crease to help remove weight from the hands.

COMING OUT On an exhalation, slowly lower your spine to the floor. Adopt the Prone Savasana position by turning your head to the right and placing your right ear where your nose was. Extend your arms along the sides of your body, palms up, and allow your legs to rotate internally, relaxing with toes in and heels out. Take two breaths and set up for a second set. At the end of the second set, relax again in Prone Savasana, this time with your left ear on the mat.

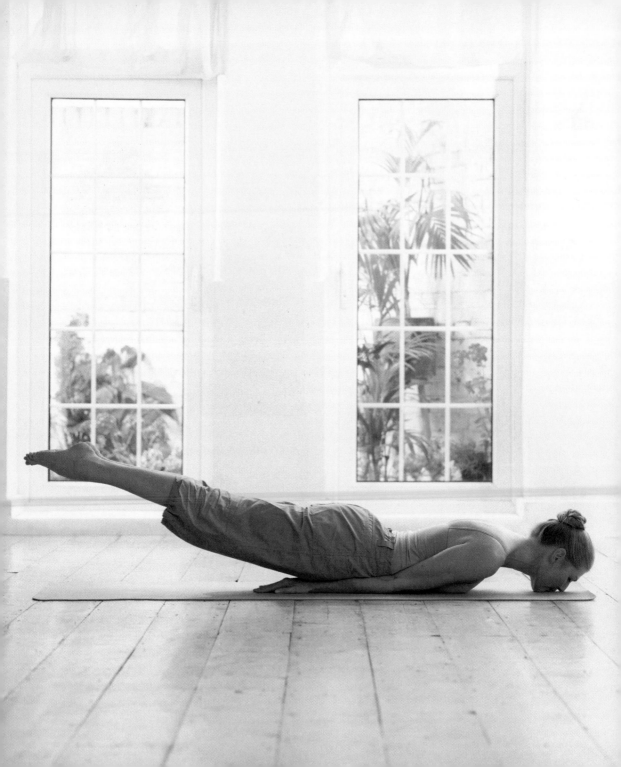

HALF-LOCUST POSE

SALABHASANA

The previous floor pose strengthened the lower spine while lifting and opening the upper body. This pose, named for *salabha,* the locust, does the opposite, strengthening the upper body while you lift and lengthen the lower body. Here, the arms are planted beneath the body, palms, wrists and elbows open to the floor. In the beginning, this can prove the greatest challenge–it feels as if your arms might break –but it is actually beneficial for those with symptoms of carpal tunnel syndrome and tennis elbow. As the palms, wrists and elbows stretch open, discomfort eases and you increase your focus on lifting into the pose. There are two parts to the pose. First, you lift one leg, then the other, the rest of the body stabilised on the floor. This stretches open the front of the pelvis, groin and front of the legs. In the second part, you lift the pelvis and legs. The upper spine draws down into the chest; the lower body lightens and lifts. Visualise a seesaw: as you add weight to one end, the other end rises.

STARTING POSITION: *lying face down, head towards the mirror.*

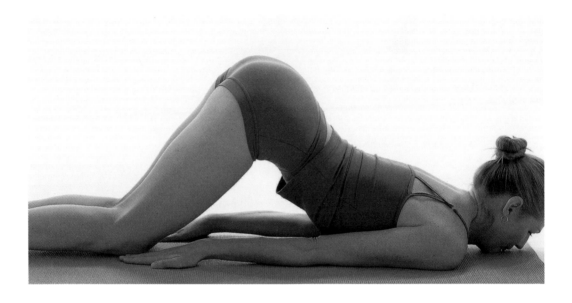

SETTING UP Turn your head to rest your nose and the front of your chin lightly on the floor. Your arms stay at your sides, inner forearms and palms facing down. Inhale space into your chest, stretching from ribs to upper arms. Rotate your inner elbows down into the floor and spiral your upper arms away to open the shoulders. Exhale and relax the upper spine down, bringing your chest to rest on the floor between your arms. Keeping your chest open into the floor, inhale and lift into the groin crease as you walk your knees in beneath your hips to raise your abdomen and pelvis off the floor. Keep your palms open to the floor, middle fingers aligned with the centre of the wrists.

Spread your fingers and thumbs apart, and slide your hands towards the centre, bringing your little fingers to touch if possible. Lie your body on your arms, flattening them out as you stretch your legs straight back on to the floor. Do not roll your shoulders in beneath the chest to bring your arms under your body; the chest stays open wide between the arms, and the arms angle in to form a triangular base.

Hot tips Palms and forearms face up? Shoulders roll under your body and chest lifts from the floor? Review your setup. Some teachers advise the following maneu-vre: roll up to one side and place that arm on the front of the body, palm up; then roll down and up to the other side to position the second arm; roll back down, lying on both arms. A tight chest is more likely to remain closed, however, when the arms are positioned in this way.

Elbows point out from your sides or won't straighten? Separate your hands enough to pull your inner elbows down into the floor, spiraling your upper arms away while drawing your chest down between your arms. Eventually work your hands back in, bringing your elbows beneath your body.

1 Lift alternate legs

Stabilise your torso to establish foundation– as your back relaxes down, gravity stretches your front open, arms straight. Keeping your torso square and slightly down, lift the right leg away from the floor, pelvis equally weighted right to left. Without pulling the leg away from the hip joint, straighten and square the right leg and foot: draw up from the knee, pull in the outer ankle, flex the toes, press out through the ball of the foot. Maintaining the stable torso and straight leg, inhale and internally rotate the thigh; exhale and lift the inside edge of the foot to raise the leg. Work breath by breath for three cycles, raising the leg as if placing the foot on the ceiling. Exhale, slowly lower. Relax the leg; repeat on the left.

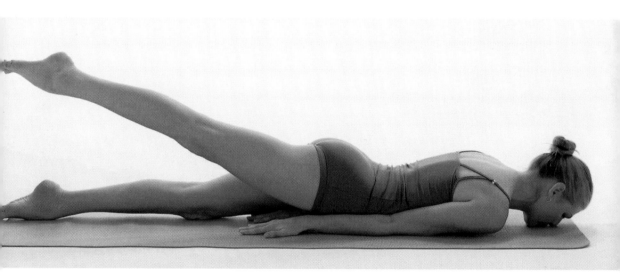

2 Lift both legs

Adjust your upper body and arms, if necessary, and keep your face down towards the mat to avoid straining your neck. (Do not lift your head to look in the mirror.) Draw your navel towards your spine and keep your sides long from ribs to hips to stabilise the middle and lower back. Bring your legs together, pulling the outer ankles in so the inner ankles and feet touch, then straighten the legs, lifting your feet from the floor. Keep the legs level with the pelvis, the body stable from crown to toes, resting on your chest, forearms and hands. Inhaling, press the back of your forearms and hands down, draw your upper spine down between your arms, and the top of your thighs towards the floor while lifting your pelvis away from your arms and hands. Focus on maintaining a stable line from lower ribs to toes; try to avoid collapsing into the lower spine.

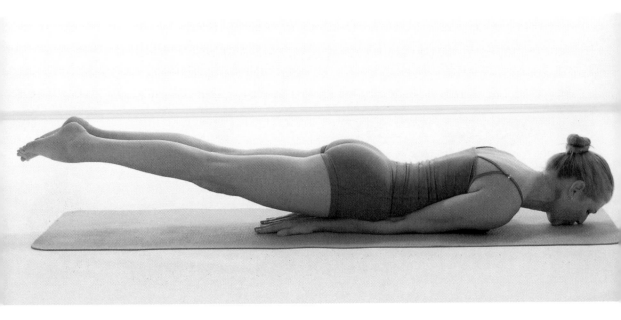

WORKING THE POSE To work with the breath, inhale and draw down into your foundation–upper back, forearms and hands–while stretching your pelvis evenly away from your ribs and up from your arms with straight legs. On each exhalation, relax your chest open to the floor and lengthen the front of your body in a straight line from ribs to toes. As the lift continues upwards, begin to feel the weight come down into the centre of your chest.

Hot tips Collapse into the lumbar spine when lifting both legs? This also happens when you try to lift the legs rather than the pelvis. In both cases, lower your legs and stabilise from ribs to toes in a straight line. (Lengthen between rib cage and pelvis, navel in, top of thighs down, top of feet up.)

COMING OUT Stabilise your foundation on an inhalation and slowly lower your body back down on the exhalation. Adopt the Prone Savasana position, turning your head to the right and relaxing for two complete breaths. Repeat a second set, then relax again in Prone Savasana, this time with your left ear on the mat.

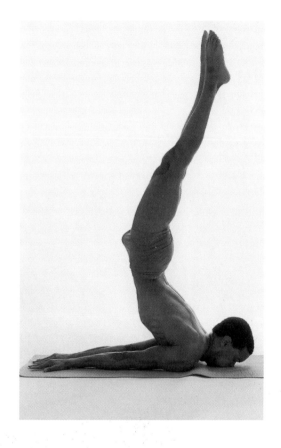

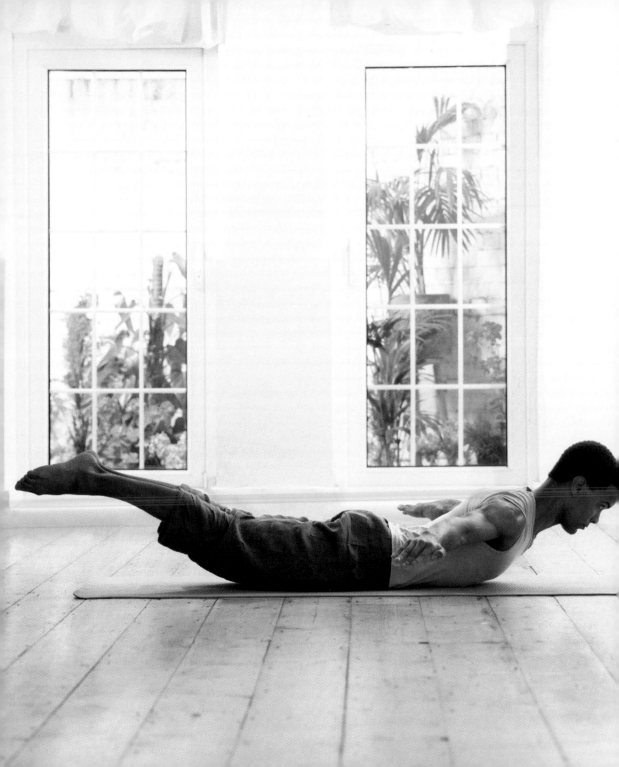

FULL LOCUST POSE

POORNA-SALABHASANA

In Sanskrit, *poorna* means full, indicating a more intense Locust Pose that strengthens the middle part of the spine. Your aim is to hold your spine in neutral and your legs straight while trying to come up into a wide 'V' shape. This requires you to lengthen both the upper and lower spine, and to stabilise in the middle where these two opposite curvatures meet–no mean feat. The lifting of the legs also stretches open the groin and strengthens the hamstrings. In a class, this pose is held for 10 seconds. Keep this length of time as your goal, bearing in mind that it may take some weeks or months of yoga practice to achieve the ideal.

STARTING POSITION: *lying face down, head towards the mirror*

SETTING UP Turn your head to bring your nose and the front of your chin to the mat. Extend your arms, palms facing down and back, approximately 15-20 cm (6-8 inches) from your hips. Stretch open the chest cavity with your breath, then exhale and relax the upper spine down, resting your chest on the floor. Do not allow your shoulders to round back down towards the floor. Bring your legs together, drawing the outer ankles in and touching the inside edge of the feet together. Firm up the legs and rotate them externally, then lift them slightly from the floor.

Next firm the arms, lifting them to shoulder–level and stabilising. Then lift your face straight up from the floor to align and stabilise the neck in a neutral position. At the same time, draw your navel up towards your spine. With the joints in the ankles, knees, wrists, elbows, shoulders and neck now stabilised, inhale, drawing into these stabilised areas and exhale, releasing any excess tension or gripping (including tension in the mind).

Hot tips When externally rotating your legs, feel your buttocks come together, firming the tailbone down towards the pubis. This is very important in stabilising the spine. If the tailbone lifts, you compress the lumbosacral region, and any effort to go up comes from the lower back (see page 23).

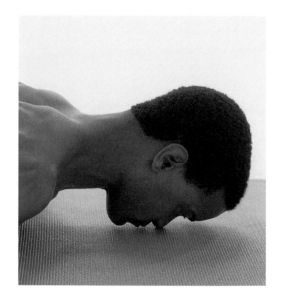

1 Raise the thighs

Imagine your calves are heavy and, on an inhalation, lift your thighs to a comfortable edge. Keep your legs together and try to open the space at the back of the knees and front of the ankles-a sensation like opening your eyes wide. Exhale, stabilise the lift and release excess tension.

Hot tips Knees bend and legs separate at the knees? Return to setting up and reestablish straight legs. In the beginning you may need to work with legs hip-width apart. To connect with the movement, practice lifting the legs only, imagining the calves are so heavy they cannot rise without the thighs.

2 Lift the upper body

Imagine the back of your head and upper back are heavy and, on an inhalation, lift the lower ribs up (not forwards and up, just up away from the floor). Continue working with the breath, coming up evenly. Work to keep the head, hands and feet at the same level, treating the entire body as two very stable pieces that 'V' upwards. Inhale to lift, and, on the exhalation, release unnecessary tension and gripping. Try to hold the pose for 10 seconds.

Hot tips   Upper back arches? Lumbar spine collapses? Lower your head, chest and arms. Stabilise this zone, keeping torso, head and arms on the same plane; lift again. Imagine the head, arms and upper back are so heavy they cannot rise above the abdomen and pelvis. Head and hands higher than feet? Bring the chest down until the head and arms are even with the feet. Continue lifting both ends equally.

COMING OUT   To release, slowly lower both parts of the 'V' to the floor on an exhalation. Adopt the Prone Savasana position, turning your head to the right and relaxing briefly. Repeat a second set, then relax again in Prone Savasana, this time with your left ear on the mat.

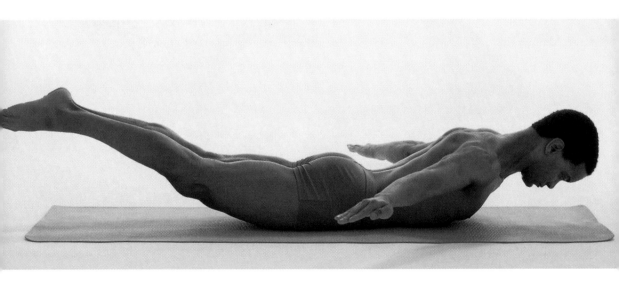

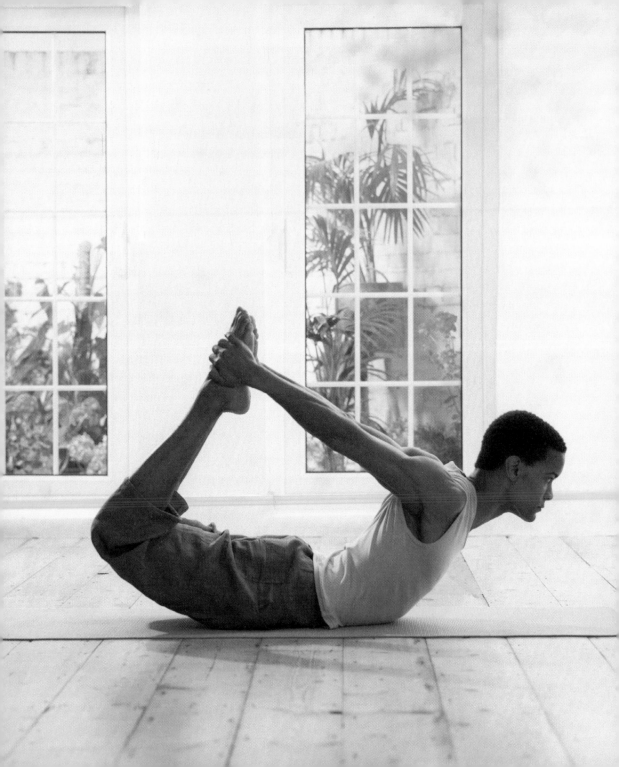

BOW POSE

DHANURASANA

Resembling a strung archer's bow in form (*dhanura* means bow), this floor pose manipulates every segment of the spine to create all the openings your body requires to achieve safe and comfortable backward bending. When performed correctly, the posture stretches the chest, groin and thighs simultaneously. Aim to hold this pose for twice as long as the previous three spine-strengthening poses, building up slowly to the 20 seconds the asana is allotted within a classroom setting.

STARTING POSITION: *lying face down, head towards the mirror.*

SETTING UP Turn your head back to centre, nose and front of chin towards the mat to keep your head and neck in the neutral position. Extending your arms down the sides of the body, palms downward, allow your inner elbows to relax towards the floor and your upper arms away. This rotation opens the chest and allows the upper spine to drop. Relax your spine down through the centre of your body. Draw your outer ankles in and point your toes away from your knees to align each foot with its leg. Engage the thighs to stabilise the knee joints, then rotate the entire leg externally. This stabilises the dropped sacrum–feel the front of the pelvis ground down towards the mat.

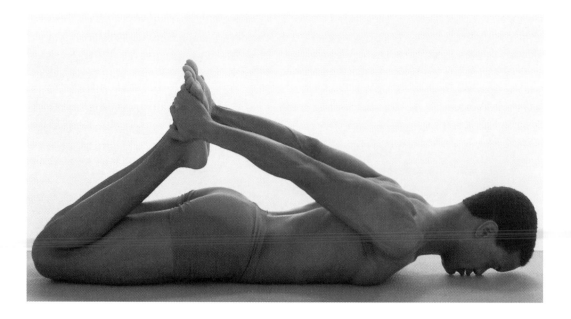

1 Establish a foundation

Fold in behind the knees and bring your heels towards your buttocks. Reach back and take hold of the outside edge of your feet, placing your palms on the sides of your feet, your fingers across the top of each foot. Flex your toes back towards your hands, then draw the ankles and lower legs in towards each other. Ideally, the legs stay hip-width and parallel, and eventually they touch. Kick your feet back to stretch your arms without lifting your body from the floor.

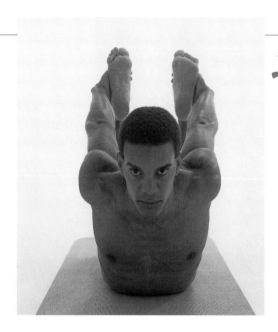

2 Lift up

Stabilise your spine down towards the floor and lift your knees. As your thighs begin to stretch upwards, keep kicking back into your hands. Lift your face and chest upwards, and arch the upper back by moving the spine forwards into your chest. Continue working with the breath, forming an archer's bow with your body. Inhale space into your chest, groin and thighs and, as you exhale, press down and stretch up. For full backbend stretching, your shoulders and knees must rise to the same level. Hold the pose for twice as long as the previous three poses–aim for 20 seconds. To avoid struggling as you hold, grow into the pose with each breath.

Hot tips Tailbone lifting the pelvis away from the floor, compressing the lower back? Release the pose enough to set the pelvis down, and begin again. Try to keep the area from groin to ribs down-take only the thighs, chest, and head up.

Knees lower than shoulders? You won't stretch evenly– the chest gets more of a stretch than the groin or thighs. Lower your chest and focus on lifting your knees. When the knees reach the height of the shoulder joint, begin again to work the stretch evenly.

Be careful not to let your head and neck hang forwards. When arching the lower back, drop the chin slightly and lift up into the crease at the throat, behind the ears and into the base of the skull. At the same time, relax your shoulders away from the ears. Now bring your face and shoulders back as the spine stretches forwards into your chest.

COMING OUT Release on an exhalation and slowly lower your body, releasing your hands from your feet. Continue releasing the legs, chest and arms down to the mat. Adopt the Prone Savasana position with your right ear down, and relax for two full breath cycles. Repeat a second set, and relax again in Prone Savasana, this time with your left ear on the mat.

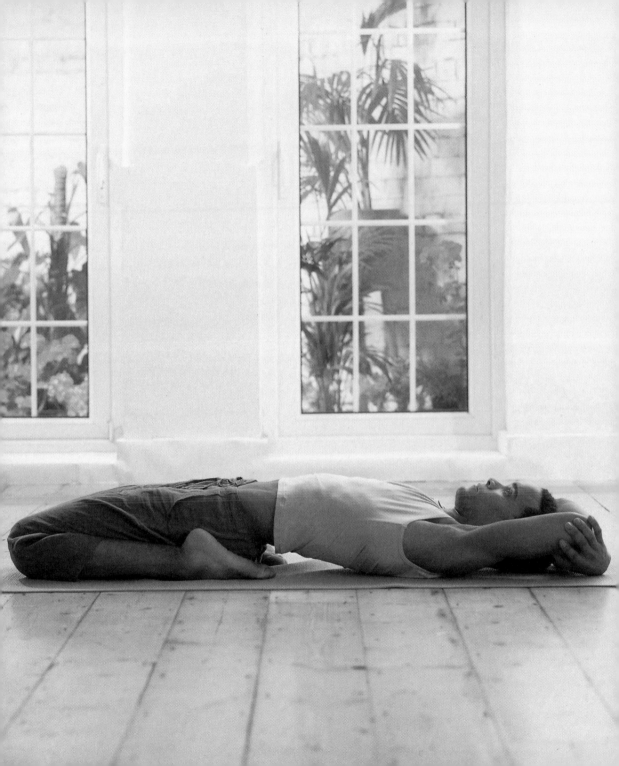

FIXED FIRM POSE

SUPTA VAJRASANA

With this pose begins a series of four postures that alternate backward and forward bending to improve spinal flexibility. In Supta Vajrasana (*supta* means between and *vajra* fixed or firm), the lower body is prepared for bending backward as you sit with legs folded between the feet, then lie back with arms overhead, grasping opposite elbows. Your focus for Fixed Firm Pose is to stretch the front of the thighs and groin–a region often neglected during back-bends. When these zones are tight, back-bending begins in the lumbar spine, creating compression to an area that naturally has less space. As you begin to rotate the pelvis back to bring the spine down to the floor, the stretch increases in the front of the leg between the knee and top of the pelvis. When performed correctly, the pose is great for rehabilitating the knees, but done incorrectly, it can create or exacerbate a knee problem. Props, such as a block or folded blanket, are very useful for those with extremely tight legs or injuries that prevent deep knee-bending.

STARTING POSITION: *kneeling at the front of mat, facing the mirror.*

SETTING UP From Prone Savasana, look down at the mat, place your hands beneath your shoulders, palms down, and turn the top of your feet down. As you press through your hands and knees, lift up your pelvis and stretch up and back through the groin crease, bringing your sitting bones back. Keep your chest, face and palms down while lifting the arms. Take a breath or two, then lift your chest and move forwards, coming on to hands and knees. Move your knees to the front edge of the mat.

Place your knees directly beneath your hips, ankles straight back from the knees, top of the feet flat. Begin to fold back at the knee joints, lowering your thighs on to your calves, and with a slight internal rotation of your folded legs, sit between your feet. The ankles and heels should touch the upper thigh: make sure there is no space between leg and hip. If you cannot sit between your feet, use a prop (see page 32).

Hot tips It's OK to let the upper legs open wider, but you must keep lower and upper legs touching. It's very bad for the knees to separate them. If this happens, come on to the knees and reposition the legs before folding at the knee. Try internally rotating and 'V'ing out the legs to get down with lower and upper legs connected. As you gain flexibility, bring the legs in and rotate them externally, lower legs pulled into upper legs.

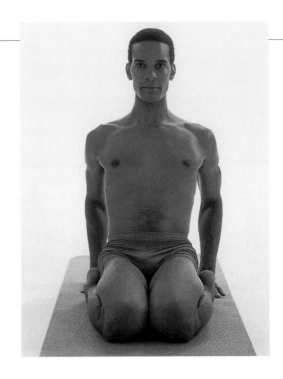

1 Begin to stretch

To stretch between the knees and top of the pelvis, place your palms on your feet, fingers towards toes. Begin to rotate the folded legs externally, turning the pelvis back. The buttocks slide underneath, the tailbone moves towards the knees, the top of the pelvis drops back towards the floor. Stretch back into the elbow creases, bending the arms and lowering right, then left elbows for support. Stabilise the spine and move the torso as one piece as far as possible. Eventually, the centre of the buttocks rest on the floor when you lie back, as shown on page 116.

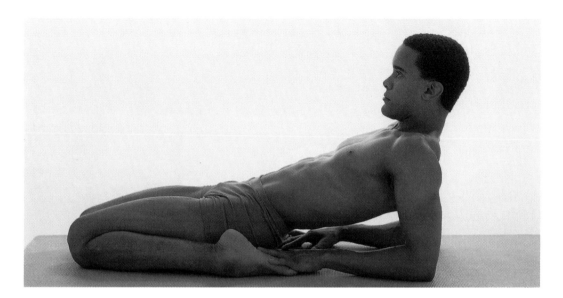

Hot tips Spine arches away from the floor? Bring the head and shoulders up to a point at which you can neutralise the spine; go back down by rotating the pelvis. Keep working the stretch in the legs and pelvis. Don't begin bending in the lower back; this stops the thighs and pelvis from stretching, and stretches the lower abdominal muscles as the lumbar spine compresses.

2 Soften the spine
Once you are lying back, use your breath to neutralise the spine. Create a soft space in the lumbar and cervical regions: inhale, opening the chest and lengthening between the knees and hip crest; exhale, relaxing your back ribs, buttocks and folded legs down to the floor.

3 Take the arms back
Bring your arms overhead without arching away from the floor. Place your hands on opposite elbows and relax as you lower the arms back into the floor. Breathe and enjoy. Aim to hold the pose for 10 seconds.

COMING OUT Come up just as you went down: bring your arms back to your sides and lift up on to the elbows, then the hands. Bringing the pelvis back over the tops of the legs, come up to sitting. Turn around and lie back in Savasana for two complete breaths. Sit up (see page 27) and turn around. Repeat a second set.

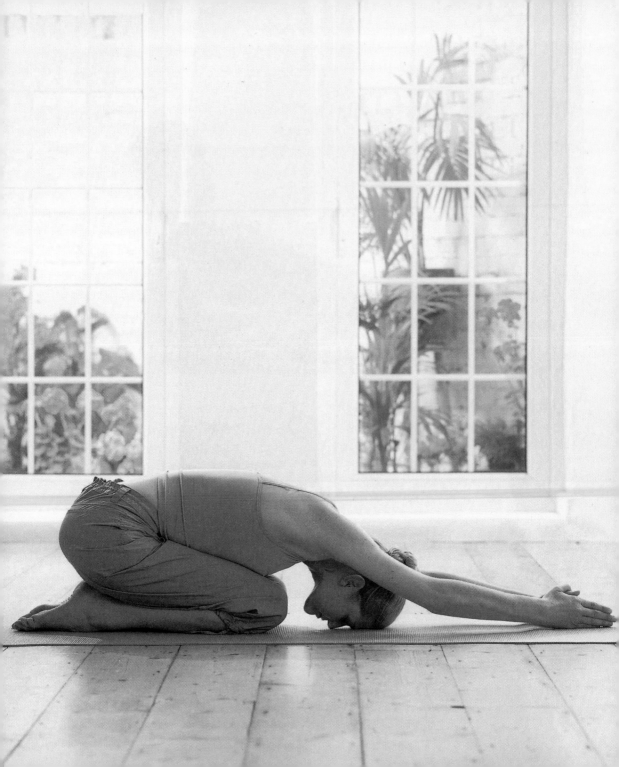

HALF-TORTOISE POSE

ARDHA-KURMASANA

You are required to sit with deeply folded legs in this floor pose. First, certain muscles in the legs have to stretch, then gravity assists you into position. Holding this folded-leg position isolates the stretch so that it becomes your foundation. Half-Tortoise Pose (*ardha* means half, *kurma* tortoise) is a forward bend with tightly folded legs, in which your focus should be on stretching the back of the thighs, buttocks and lower back. You sit on the heels with legs and feet pulled together, arms extended overhead with hands in prayer position and pelvis rotated forwards to bring the spine over the thighs. The forehead and sides of the little fingers rest on the floor. It is important to stabilise the spine in a neutral position and to move the pelvis to bring it over the legs. This gives you maximum stretch in the areas that require it.

STARTING POSITION: *on hands and knees at the front of the mat, facing the mirror.*

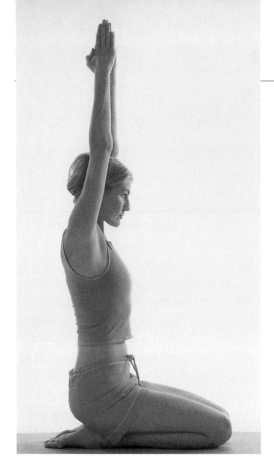

Create a foundation

Inhale into the groin crease and feel your legs firm up, then draw your legs down to begin creating a foundation. As you exhale, stabilise the legs and begin to rotate your pelvis forwards. Keep the front of your body open (creating a long, straight line between groin crease and top of the forehead) as you take your spine down over your legs (see forward bending, page 24).

SETTING UP On hands and knees, bring your legs together, heels touching, top of the feet down. Sit on your heels with an upright spine. Inhale and take your arms overhead, hands in prayer position with thumbs crossed. Exhale and relax the front of the thighs down to stabilise your body as you lengthen up, opening the front of the body and relaxing your shoulders over your hips.

Hot tips Unable to sit on your heels? Use a block, folded towel, or blanket to provide support.

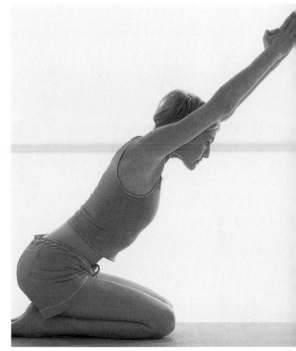

2 Take the head down

Once your body is laid on top of your thighs, allow your head to come down, placing your nose and forehead on the mat. Then take the side of your hands down and draw your forearms in, straightening the wrists and elbows. Take the sides of the little fingers down and move your shoulders away from your ears. Try to hold the pose for 10 seconds, as in a class.

Hot tips If, when coming down from the groin crease over the thighs, you find yourself closing the 'V' without rounding forwards, you might need to keep your arms at your sides until your chest and upper spine are down. At this point, bring your arms overhead, hands in prayer position with thumbs crossed, and finish setting up. When you release, you may need to take your arms to the side before coming up to sitting. As your strength and flexibility begin to balance, you will be able to take the arms back overhead.

WORKING THE POSE Use your breath in the pose to inhale space into the back of the thighs, buttocks and lower back. Exhale down into the folds of the legs and relax the spine down into the front of the body.

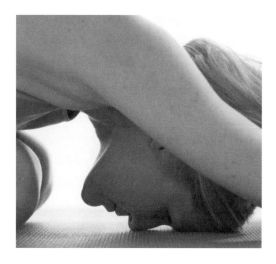

COMING OUT To release, inhale, lifting the head, neck and chest up enough to neutralise the spine. Exhale and stabilise the spine while lifting the sides of the little fingers off the mat. Inhaling, rotate the pelvis away from the thighs, bringing your spine upright with arms overhead. Exhale and take your arms down to your sides. Turn around and lie back in Savasana for two complete breaths, then do a Sit-Up (see page 27) and turn around. Repeat a second set.

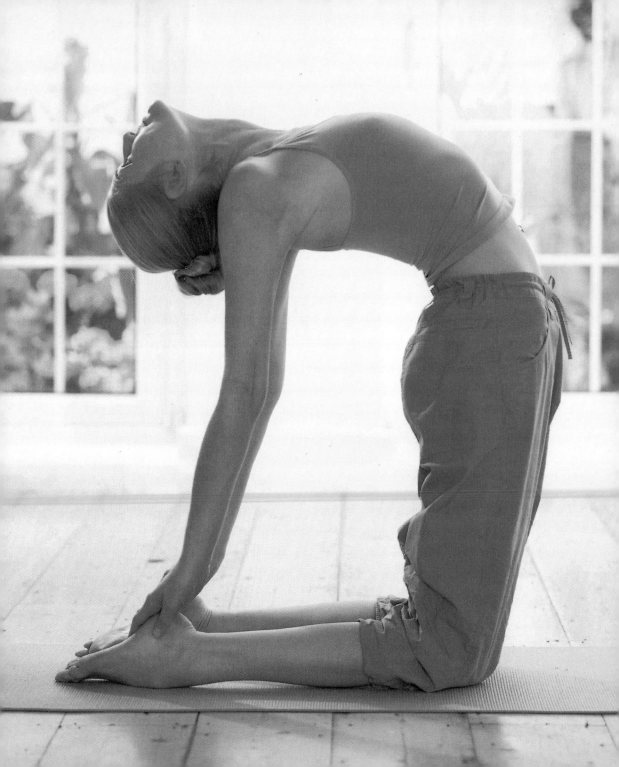

CAMEL POSE

USTRASANA

The previous two floor postures comprised backward and forward bends in which movement was initiated in the lower portion of the torso, and your primary focus was the legs and hips. During the next two postures, movement begins in the upper portion of the torso, and your focus turns to the neck, chest and abdomen. In Camel Pose you stand on your knees, arch your upper spine, reach back to grab the heels and lift your spine to stretch open the chest. The throat and abdomen also benefit from the intense stretch.

STARTING POSITION: *kneeling at the front of the mat, facing the mirror.*

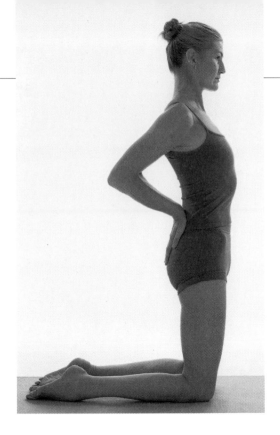

SETTING UP Kneel upright with legs hip-width apart: hips over knees; lower legs and feet (toes pointing away) directly behind the knees. Let the back of your lower legs and feet move towards the floor to form the foundation from which you rise up. Relax your tailbone down, and move the back of the thighs and buttocks forwards as you stretch up the front of the legs to the top of the pelvis, stabilising the legs and hips above the knee. Extend your arms down your sides, rotated so palms face forwards.

1 Take back the palms

Inhale and lift your forearms, drawing back through your elbow creases to take your hands behind your hips. Drop your hands without moving your forearms, and place your palms on your buttocks, fingers pointing down, thumbs to the side. Exhale, stabilising into your foundation as the front of your body lengthens from crown to knees.

Hot tips Keep the body, including your head, upright when pulling your arms back; feel your spine begin to lengthen forwards into your chest.

2 Bend back the upper spine

Inhaling, draw down into your foundation and hold the back of the body forwards as you bring space with the breath into your front. At the same time, start bending back from beneath the shoulder blades, spine lifting into the chest and neck. The back of the head moves back and down with the upper spine (chin relaxed to the throat). Exhale, stabilising the back. Form a long line from base of shoulder blades to back of knees as you lengthen your front over the supported arch. Lengthen the back of the neck, shoulders rolling away from ears.

3 Take hands to heels

Working with the breath, release your right palm from your buttock and move it back as you straighten the arm and reach down to your right heel. Cup the heel with your palm, thumb on the outside. Then lift along your right side, holding the heel, and release your left palm. Move it back and reach down for your left heel. Lift your spine as you pull on the heels, move your chin away from your throat, and allow your head to hang back from the neck. Work with the pose for 10 seconds.

Hot tips Can't reach back for the heels without collapsing the lower back? Keep hands on hips and work on developing the upper-back arch, using the arms for support. Press through the base of the palms while drawing back into the elbow creases to lift the base of the shoulder blades, taking the upper spine back and down. Bring chin to throat while lengthening the back of the neck to keep the head supported and stop the cervical spine from collapsing. Open the spine in the chest and back of neck before dropping the head.

WORKING THE POSE Open the chest with the breath by lifting and lengthening the upper spine into the strong arch. Inhale, draw the tailbone down and anchor the lower legs, then lengthen the lower and middle spine up while expanding the chest. Exhale; lift upper spine into chest as you pull on the heels.

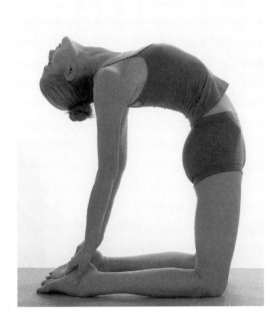

COMING OUT Come up the way you went down, with support. Inhale, lift up into the spine and release your right, then left hands to reach up for the hips. Continue lifting your spine up and forwards to upright. Exhale your arms down to your sides, and sit back on your heels for one breath. Turn around and lie back in Savasana for two complete breaths. Perform a Sit-Up, turn around and repeat a second set.

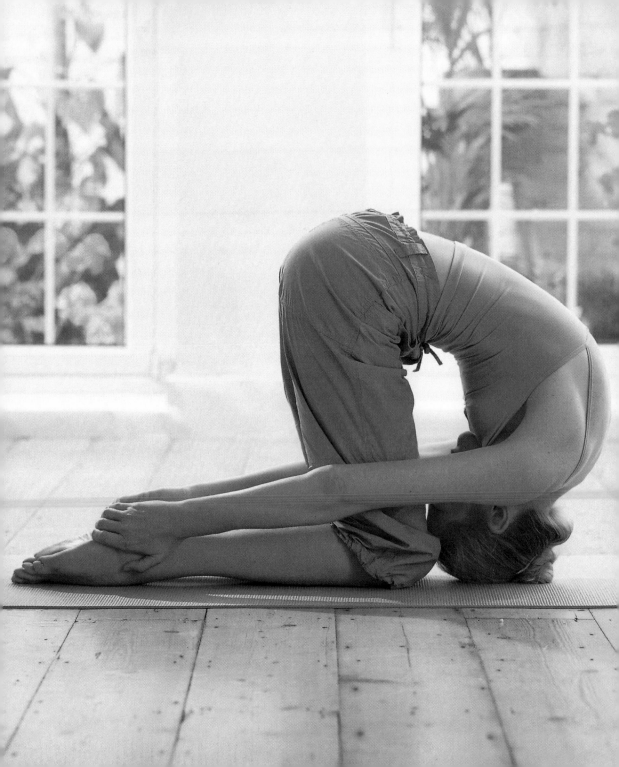

RABBIT POSE

SASANGASANA

This pose is another forward bend in which the spine is rounded with forehead on the knee (*sasa* means hare, or moon; *samga* closing or coming together). Here, you sit on the heels, tuck forehead to knees and lift the hips, rolling forwards as if attempting a somersault while holding the heels until the arms extend fully, hips over knees. Your focus is continually to lift your spine through the abdomen and take the shoulders away from the ears to prevent head and neck compression. Rabbit Pose opens every posterior vertebral joint while stretching the sides, back of the neck and lower back. Deep compression to the throat and upper abdomen stimulates glands and vital organs. As always, begin lengthening areas of the spine that naturally bend back, so the entire spine stretches without stressing those segments at which the curvature changes. In Rabbit Pose, this approach is even more important because of your change in foundation: when upside-down, it is all too easy to let gravity take you forwards via the path of least resistance.

STARTING POSITION: *sitting on your heels at the front of the mat, facing the mirror.*

SETTING UP Sit up on your heels with heels together (draw the outer ankles in; stretch out through the big toes to pull the feet together). Keep your arms at your sides. Rotate your arms open and take them back towards your hips as you tilt forwards from the hips. Inhale, bringing your chin into your throat without tilting your head forwards or collapsing the chest. Exhale, tilting your head forwards while taking the shoulders away from the ears. Inhaling, take the lower ribs back, lifting the abdomen in and up while pulling the tops of the thighs back to lengthen the lumbar spine.

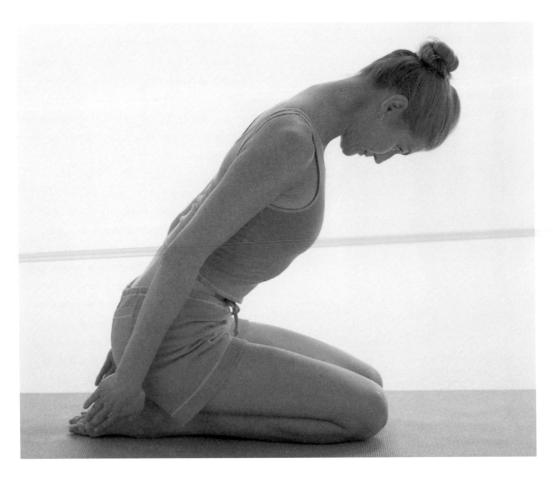

Hot tips Unable to keep your heels together and the tops of your feet on the mat? Come on to your knees to reposition the feet. Place your knees so your thighs are parallel, lower legs aligned directly behind the knees. Straighten out each foot to align with the leg by pulling the ankle in while stretching in behind the inner knee crease as the toes extend evenly away from the knee. Place the top of each ankle and foot on the mat, then, without releasing the ankles, bring your legs together and sit down. Feel a slight internal rotation. Keeping the front of the ankle opened into the floor creates a strong foundation; without this anchor, you cannot lift the hips to roll forwards with control. Most people habitually sit on the feet with toes in and heels out. This overstretches the outer ankle and foot and shortens the inner side, making full extension of the front of the ankle difficult.

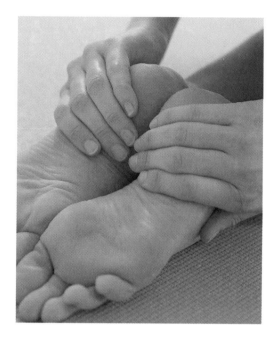

1 Forehead to knees
Contract your chest, rounding your upper back to kiss your forehead against your knees. As you are doing this, rotate your forearms to turn your palms towards the side of your heels, placing your fingers over the heels and your thumbs along the side of the foot to hold on to the feet. Hold the ankles in and keep pressing the tops of the feet and ankles down to provide your foundation.

2 Roll forwards

Keeping your forehead kissing the knees and your hands on your feet, inhale, anchoring into your foundation and expanding the back of your body with the breath. Exhale, lift your hips and roll forwards until your arms are fully extended while lifting your shoulders and spine to keep weight from shifting forwards on to your head. Ideally, the hips are directly above the knees, as shown on page 128. Continue to open up the inner circle you have formed against the backside of the body, creating a wheel shape. Work with the breath for 20 seconds.

Hot tips If you are unable to bend forwards and reach your heels, perhaps because of your weight, use the instructions for the modified pose.

COMING OUT On an exhalation, lower your thighs down to your heels and release your chin from your throat. Inhaling, draw the front of the body back and up as you unroll, stacking the vertebrae to sit in an upright position. Take a breath here before turning around to lie back in Savasana for two complete breaths. Perform a Sit-Up, turn around and repeat a second set.

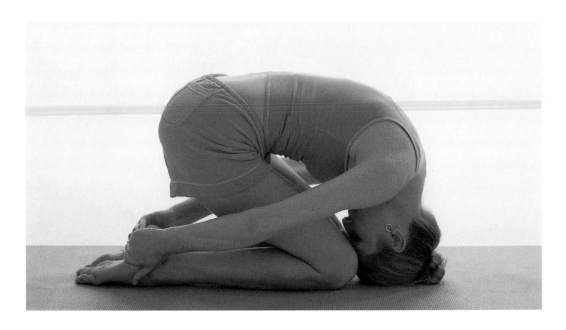

Modified stretch

Start on hands and knees with legs together (ankles in, inner edges of feet touching, tops of feet and ankles open to the mat). Bring the thighs forwards, hips over knees. Place the base of the palms under the shoulders, middle fingers centred, fingers wide; press down evenly. Keep the face parallel to the floor, shoulders away from ears. Fold the elbows, lower elbows behind wrists, bringing your forearms to the mat. Inhale the chin into the throat without tilting the head or collapsing the chest. Exhale, tilt the head forwards, and lift beneath the crease of the throat while moving shoulders away from ears. Inhale the lower ribs towards the spine without rounding the upper back, and lift the abdomen in and up while stretching into the groin crease. Stabilise lower legs, ankles and tops of feet down. As you bring sitting bones away from heels, contract chest, round upper back and place crown between elbows. Lift into the throat and abdomen, moving shoulders away from ears by pressing the forearms. Maintain the foundation in the lower legs and forearms. To release, take chin from throat, and lengthen throat, chest and pelvis. Press on the palms to lift the spine parallel to the floor as the elbows straighten. Lower sitting bones to heels; walk the hands back to sit upright.

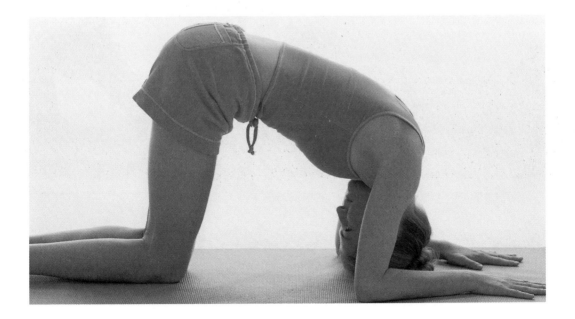

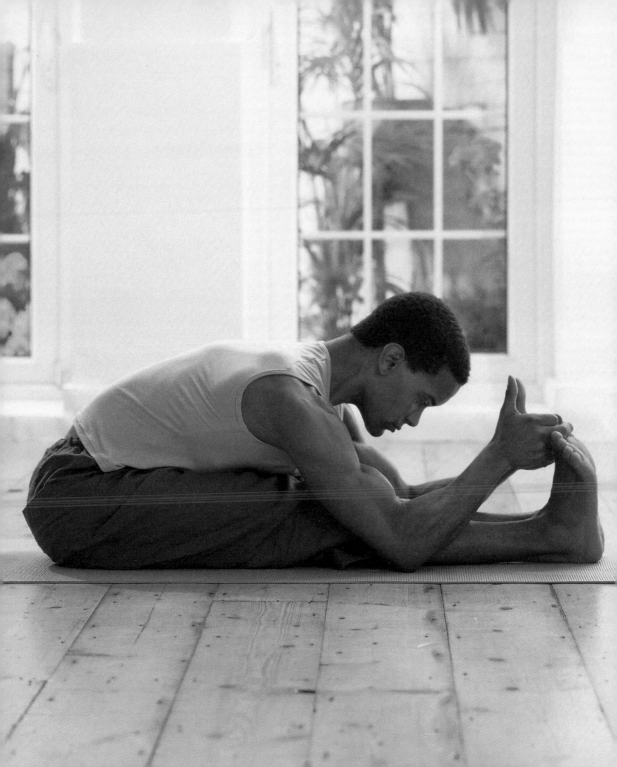

HEAD-TO-KNEE POSE WITH STRETCHING POSE

JANUSHIRASANA &
PASCHIMOTTHANASANA

The penultimate floor pose has three parts and offers a wonderful combination of stretches. In the first two parts, forward bends with a spinal twist lead to rounding of the upper spine and stretching of the back of the legs. The third part comprises a full forward bend like the last part of Half-Moon Pose (pages 48-49), that weds spinal extension with a stretch to the back of the legs. In the Sanskrit, *paschima* means west, *ut* intense and *tan* extension-this is an intense stretch for the west side (back of the body). You start the pose with legs in a 'V' shape, then rotate rib cage and shoulders towards the thigh, bend the knee and flex the spine to place forehead to knee. Your focus is straightening the leg as the upper spine rotates and flexes. In the third move, aim to extend the spine fully and straighten the legs as the torso eventually connects to the front of the legs. Because most back injuries occur as a result of improper deep forward bending and twisting, take time to understand the body mechanics of the pose.

STARTING POSITION: *sitting at the centre of the mat, facing the mirror.*

SETTING UP Open your legs to create a 'V' (a 60° angle). Place your hands back towards your hips, fingers spread and pointing away, thumbs beneath hips at the groin crease. Tilt your pelvis, bringing your body forwards slightly over your thighs. Pressing down with fingers and thumbs, straighten your elbows, lifting through your chest and lightening the pelvis away from the legs. At the same time, point the toes to firm the legs and internally rotate the legs to free the pelvis. Set your legs down and bring your pelvis and body upright, tall on the sitting bones. Refirm the legs, and rotate back to centre, flexing feet and toes, knees and feet pointing up, spine rising out of the pelvis.

Bring your left knee up, heel sliding to sitting bone, calf pressing into thigh. Place your hands, fingers interlaced, below the knee, inhale and stretch into the groin crease, elbow folds and ball of the foot as your chest and knee crease rise. Exhale and anchor the left sitting bone as you relax the back of the thigh and hip down to solidify the foundation. Slide the outside edge of the left foot towards centre (foot and toes flexed) to drop the folded leg left. When the knee is almost down, keep the toes flexed and extend the ankle. To do this, point away foot, then toes to place the outside edge of the top of the foot and leg down. Bring the folded leg in close and flat (ideally, heel against body

in the centre). Bring your left big toe towards the shin as you slide your right leg over so left sole touches right inner thigh. Right leg and foot are squared, toes and foot flexed, foot and knee straight up.

Sitting tall, extend the arms, open the palms, and spread fingers and thumbs wide. Bring the arms back towards your sides, rotating externally so palms and inner elbows face out. While inhaling, press down the legs and shoulders and rise from hipbones to chest as you lift the forearms to take your arms overhead. Exhale, pull the elbows in and relax shoulders away from ears as you stabilise your foundation.

Inhale (toes and foot flexed), lift behind your right knee, and slide your right heel as far as possible towards the sitting bone without losing your foundation (sitting bones, left inner thigh, right heel). Exhale and stabilise.

Hot tips Can't sit on the sitting bones with pelvis tucked under? Place a prop beneath them (see page 32). While sitting tall, reach back and pull loose flesh out from beneath the sitting bones. When dropping the folded leg, support the outer ankle with your left hand as the knee comes down. Then inhale, lift the outer ankle and sitting bone into the body; exhale, and relax the inner leg. Feel the leg release down on the mat. Throughout the movement be aware of your foundation.

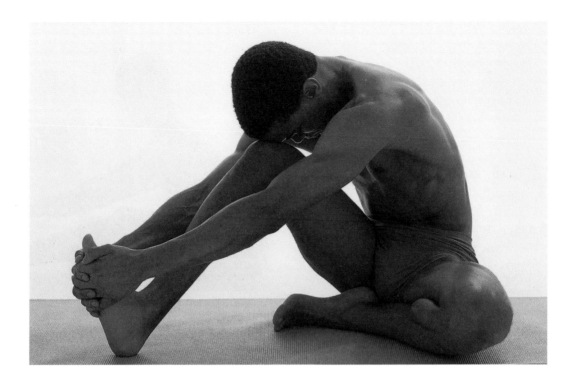

1 Rotate to the right

Carefully rotate your rib cage away from your left side so your chest and shoulders turn towards your right thigh. Inhale, lengthening your sides as you ground into your foundation and your spine rises through the centre. Exhale, looking forwards and rotate the rib cage only to the right. Take several breaths to rotate chest and shoulders, learning to isolate the move. When the chest is centred with the thigh, turn your head right to look over the knee. Inhale, bring your chin into your throat and lift under the ears and into the base of the skull as the head tilts, moving shoulders away from ears. Place forehead on knee and reach out, interlacing the hands behind the ball of the foot. Exhale into your sitting bones, up through the lower abdomen, and release into the upper-body twist. Inhale into your foundation, rising up under the ribs. Exhale, rotate your upper body, and slide heel away from sitting bone, hands interlaced behind the foot, forehead on knee.

Work with the breath until your leg is fully extended. Aim to work each segment of pose for 10 seconds.

To release, let the foot go, release the chin, bring your upper body up and twist back to centre. Pause to inhale and exhale, then release the left leg back to the 'V' formation.

✳ **Hot tips** When rotating the rib cage, look forwards to help isolate the move; watch in the mirror to see what you feel and resist any movement not consistent with your goal. The body typically follows the eyes; since you don't want anything below the ribs to follow, pay close attention to your intention.

WORKING THE POSE For advanced students, stretch into the elbow folds, bring the elbows down to the mat next to each calf and lift your right heel from the floor.

2 Work the left side
Begin the setup again, this time with right leg folded in, then reverse the directions for step 1 to stretch the other side of the body.

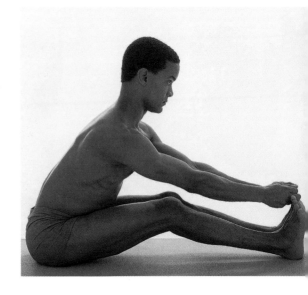

3 Connect trunk and thighs
Lie back and perform a quick Sit-Up. Turn sideways, profile in the mirror. Walk your legs back to sit on your sitting bones, and pull away loose flesh. Firm the legs; flex feet and toes. Bring the legs together and rotate them internally to touch. Lifting behind the knees and scooting heels towards sitting bones, stretch the hipbones, lower ribs and chest up the front of your legs, closing gaps from the groin crease up.

Reach forwards and place first and second fingers between first and second toes; place your thumb on top of the big toe and wrap the fingers around. Draw back through the elbow creases, open the chest and move shoulders and head back to align yourself from crown to tailbone. Inhale into the groin and ankle creases as spine and back thighs rise up into each other. Keep ears over shoulders, shoulders away from ears. Exhaling, anchor into your foundation (sitting bones and heels) as you slide the heels forwards to straighten your legs. Work with the breath until your legs are extended to the point at which you can no longer maintain both the spinal extension and connection with the thighs.

At this point, exhaling, lower the knees and bring the torso up in one piece, straightening your arms as you pull back the toes, feet fully flexed. Torso and legs form a 'V.' Work

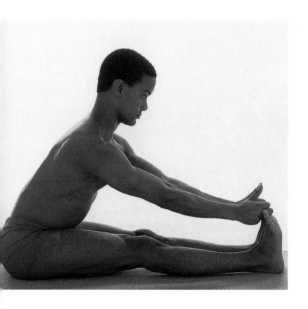

with your breath, keeping your legs firm as you continue to extend the spine over them. As you inhale, rotate the legs internally while rotating the pelvis forwards and, starting at the back of the pelvis, pull your spine up and open across the width of the chest. On the exhalation, stretch forwards through the ankle creases and stretch back into the crease of the groin and elbows, folding the body in half.

Hot tips Maintain full connection of legs and torso as in the fourth step of Half-Moon Pose (see pages 48-49). Trying to pull a rounded back over the legs is physically impossible and harmful (see page 28). Difficult to maintain even foot flexion? Outside edge of the foot stretches away? Instead of holding the big toes, place your hands on the sides of the feet to help work through inflexibilities and weaknesses in the sides of the legs and feet. Make sure to pull the outer ankle in. If your legs are straight, soften behind the knees with a slight bend, point the foot and flex the toes, keeping feet square with legs, then flex the feet.

COMING OUT Let go of your toes and lift up behind the knees, sliding your heels back while bringing your spine upright. Pause to inhale and exhale, turn around and lie back in Savasana for two complete breaths. Perform a Sit-Up, turn around, and repeat a second set.

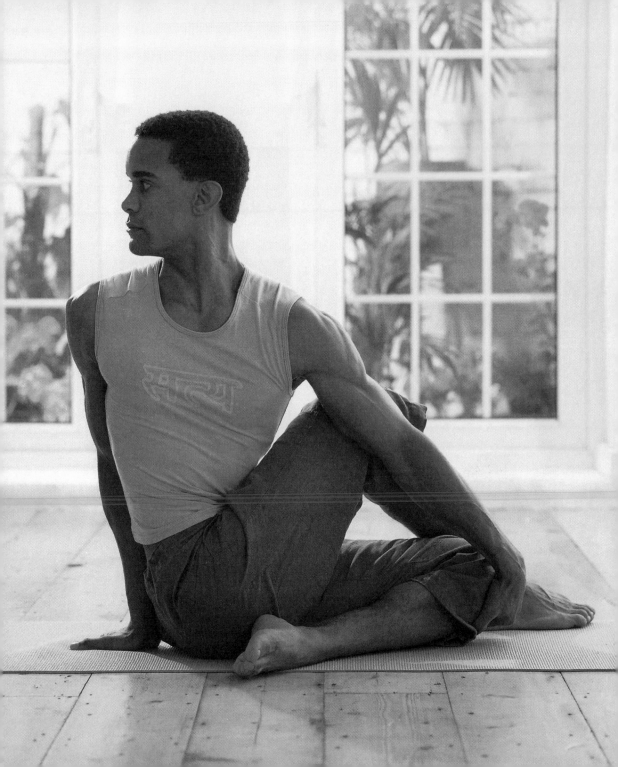

SPINE TWISTING POSE

ARDHA - MATSYENDRASANA

You have reached the final floor pose of the hot yoga series: the last exercise in the series consists of cleansing work with the breath. Spinal twisting is a neutralising move in which you work diagonally with the right and left sides of the spine. It also provides a nice massage for the internal vital organs. In this pose you remain seated with legs folded and crossed, spine upright and twisting from the bottom of the rib cage up to the skull to bring the knees and shoulders into a single line. The hips and shoulders should remain level and the spine upright. On releasing, you experience an intense sensation of refreshment, both physical and mental.

STARTING POSITION: *sitting at the centre of the mat, facing the mirror.*

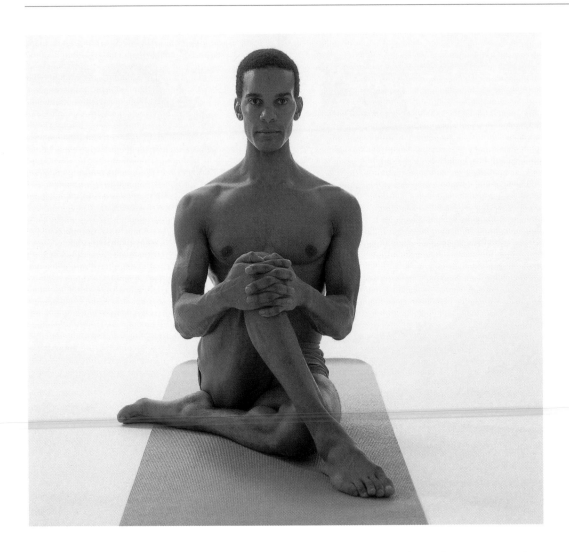

SETTING UP Sit on your sitting bones with knees bent, soles of the feet on the floor. Inhale down into your sitting bones and heels to ground the body, and on the exhalation rise up beneath the crease at the knees and underarms, relaxing the groin crease and shoulders down. Keep your ears over your shoulders, eyes looking forwards.

1 Arrange the legs

Slide your left foot up beneath your right thigh, pointing the toes evenly away from your knee to keep the ankle straight as you place the outside of the leg on the mat, heel next to the outside of the right sitting bone. Inhale into the sitting bones again, and, exhaling, rise up to lengthen both sides of your torso. Place your right leg over your left, heel by the top of the left knee. Keep both sitting bones on the mat to level the pelvis. There should be a straight line from left to right toes (left toes, heel, lower leg, knee, right heel, toes.)

Hot tips Unable to sit on both sitting bones with pelvis and shoulders level and both sides of the body equal in length? Keep your bottom leg straight and place your left heel in front of your right sitting bone with the leg straight. Bend your right leg, placing the heel on the outer side of the left knee in front of the left sitting bone. Alternatively, use props to level your hips and shoulders (see page 32). Place something beneath the sitting bone on the mat to bring it to the same level as the other. When you ground down into the prop, the other hip counterbalances, allowing a stretch down your higher side.

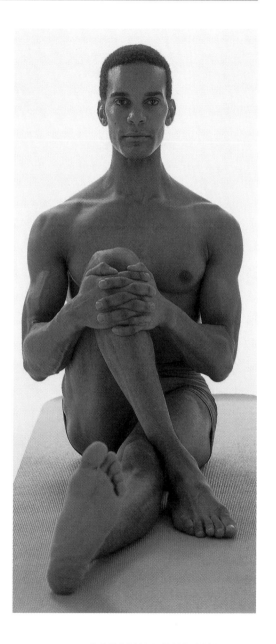

2 Twist the spine

With arms extended down, straighten from fingertips to shoulder, then rotate, palms facing up. Inhale, stretching down into the fold at the groin as the front of your torso rises and opens across the chest. Bring your right lower side and thigh into each other, your shoulders and ears away from each other. Exhale and stabilise, keeping your right lower side (below the ribs) into the thigh, your head facing forwards. Then twist your rib cage and shoulders to take the left side of the ribs to the right thigh. Keep working with your breath to rotate the chest, bringing the shoulders in line with the knee. Place the back side of your left arm on the outside of the right lower leg, then rotate the forearm to place the palm on the left knee. Rotate the right forearm to turn the palm to face left, lift up into the crease of the right elbow, then take the folded arm behind you. With the elbow below the shoulder and the forearm against the body, reach around with the hand to place the palm on the left thigh.

3 Work with the breath

Once the spinal twist is set up, bring your chin around to your right shoulder, keeping it parallel to the floor, and look to the right. Work with the breath. Inhale down into your sitting bones, and rise up through your centre, opening the front of the body; on the exhalation stabilise and twist your chest, shoulders, neck, chin and eyes, looking all the way to the right.

Modified stretches

If you cannot twist enough to place your left arm over your left leg without collapsing in the chest, lift your forearm, folding in at the elbow, and place the palm on your right knee, keeping the elbow down. Stretch into the crease of the elbow when you inhale into the groin crease.

If you are unable to reach your right arm around your back without collapsing the chest, place your palm on the floor by your hip, fingers pointing away, as shown on page 140. Press into the floor through the base of the palm when you inhale.

COMING OUT On an exhalation, turn your head back, release your right then left arms, and bring your chest back around past centre to countertwist gently to the left before resting back to centre. Release your legs and set up again, reversing the instructions to work on your left side.

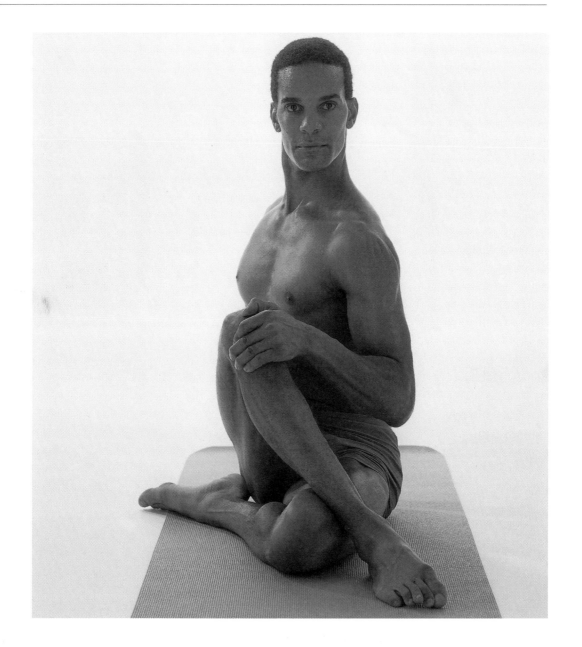

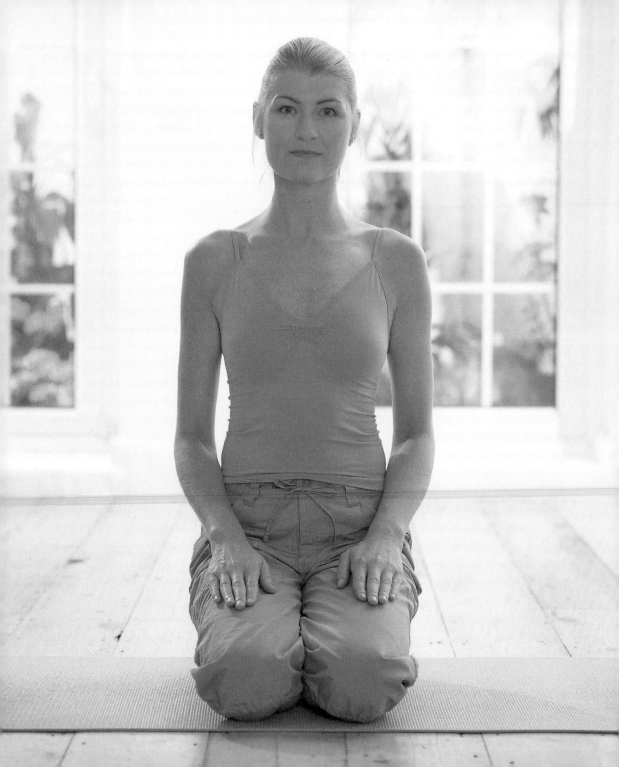

BLOWING IN FIRM (HERO) POSE

KAPALBHATI & VAJRASANA

Hot yoga begins and ends with pranayama, breathwork. At the start of the series, it opened the lung tissue, allowing more vital life-force to enter the body. This final pranayama is cleansing, removing excess carbon dioxide–a by-product of metabolism. It is performed sitting in Vajrasana, Hero Pose. The breath is an exhalation only–the abdomen contracts in and up, forcing air up and out. Inhalation comes automatically as a response to the release of the abdominal contraction, drawing air naturally back into the lungs. Although in hatha yoga this type of breathing is frequently taught through the nostrils, in hot yoga, you work 100% through the mouth. It is also known as 'skull shining' (*kapala* means skull): feel the breath come up and behind the roof of the mouth and out through the nostrils, shining the skull. The action is heat producing and stimulating, burning off and clearing mind and body of congestion or stagnation.

STARTING POSITION: *sitting at the centre of the mat.*

SETTING UP With legs together and folded, sit upright on your heels. Keep your spine upright so the joints stack: ankles beneath hips beneath shoulders, ears over shoulders. The abdomen is long, chest open, shoulders relaxed, chin parallel to the floor. Straighten your arms in front of your chest, shoulder-width apart with palms facing, and rotate them externally to set the chest in the open position. Then turn your palms down by rotating at the wrists, and set your straight arms on your thighs. Extend the arms fully, resting palms above the knee on the thighs.

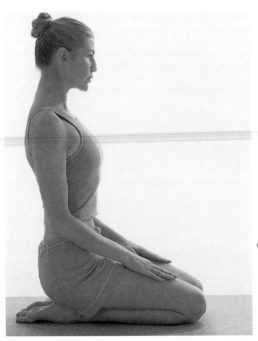

Hot tips Can't sit comfortably on your heels? Place a prop such as a folded blanket beneath your sitting bones to relieve pressure on the knees (see page 32). If you can't sit comfortably with heels together because the front of the ankle is tight, place a rolled towel or the rolled end of the mat beneath your ankles.

Spine rounds forwards when your arms are straight? Relax into the elbow creases and slide your palms up the thighs as you lengthen your belly and open your chest. Let your elbows hang below your shoulders as you hold the spine upright.

Begin the breath
Smoothly inhale and exhale completely, relaxing the mind and any gripping tension used to hold the body in position. Contract your lips in front of your teeth as if blowing up a balloon, then draw your abdomen deeply inward and up along the spine as you make a 'SHHH' sound. At the end of the sound relax your abdomen and feel the breath come back naturally into your body. Repeat for a total of 60 counts. After finishing the first set, take a full, deep inhalation and exhale completely.

Hot tips Relaxation is the key to moving the air in and out effectively and comfortably.

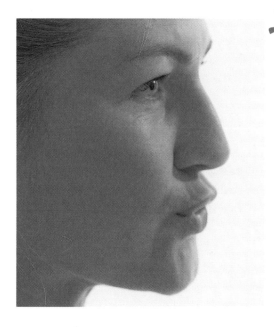

Hot tips Practice slowly and methodically until you achieve the feeling of a strong abdominal contraction and full emptying of the lungs followed by an abdominal relaxation and natural filling of the lungs.

COMING OUT When you are ready, rise up and turn around to lie on your back for the final Savasana.

2 Perform a second set

Begin a second set, making it faster this time, while retaining the same intensity of abdominal contraction. At the end of the second set, seal your practice by taking a slow, full inhalation, then make a fist with your right hand and place it at your navel, covering it with the palm of your left hand. Exhale very softly and slowly as you fold over from the hips, placing your forehead in front of your knees. Continue the very slow release of breath and body until you reach a point of stillness, and enjoy the open space you feel inside.

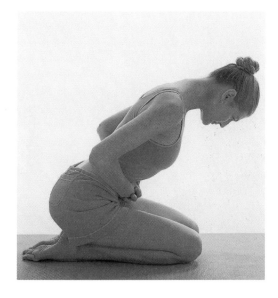

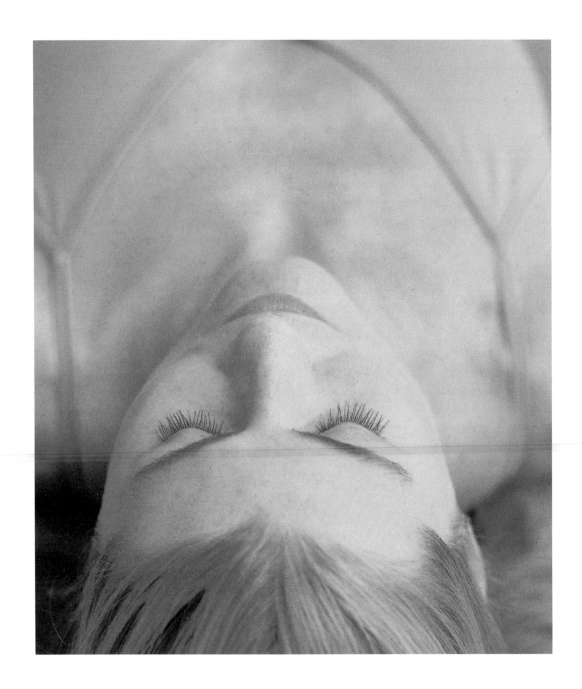

THE COOL-DOWN

To get the most out of a yoga routine, follow strenuous work on poses with these simple cool-down techniques, designed to relax mind and body and bring you back down to earth, physically and mentally. The final Savasana–the finishing touch to your routine–is one of the most important poses to follow any yoga practice. It is not unusual to drift away or briefly doze off in this posture as this is the first time you close your eyes in a pose. During the period you spend in the pose, the body is able to receive the full benefits of the time you just invested in yourself. As you completely relax, circulation flows freely into areas you have now awakened, bringing vital nourishment to cells once made stagnant by inactivity. It also gives the body a chance to transform newly created energy into stored energy for future use. The final Savasana offers the body and mind an opportunity to incorporate the new feeling of awareness you have experienced; it allows time for new patterns to become part of your physical and mental memory. For maximum benefit, please allow yourself at least five minutes to enjoy just being.

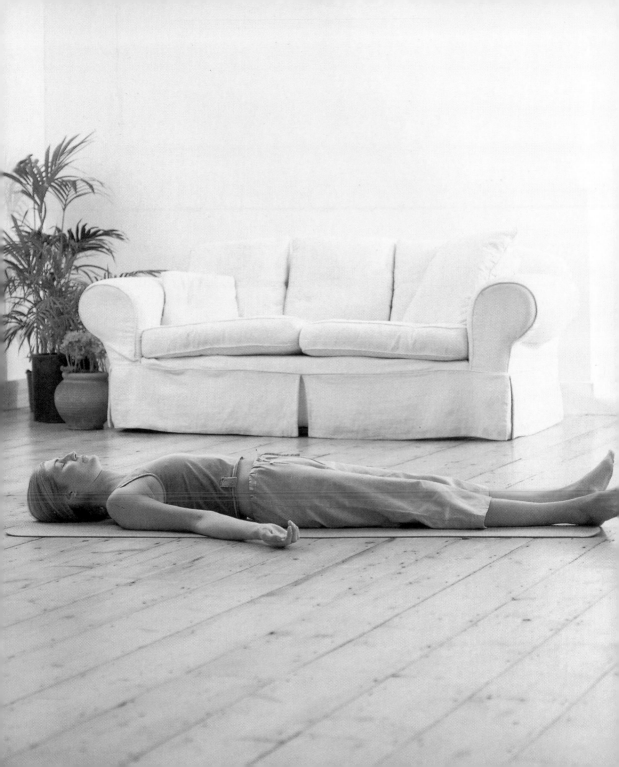

SAVASANA

FINAL DEAD BODY POSE

SAVASANA

Savasana (from the Sanskrit *sava*, meaning corpse) is one of the principal asanas in yoga. Its essence is relaxation, which relieves fatigue and promotes peace of mind. When you enter Savasana between postures in a hot yoga class, you try to get to the optimum position quickly, but during this final Savasana, take time really to establish the best possible alignment to enhance the pose. There are many ways to appreciate this asana, and they vary with the props available to you and the time allotted. Instructions follow for probably the most common basic position taught in a Bikram Method setting. In class, always lie in Savasana with your feet away from the front of the room or mirrors. A very senior teacher once told me that not pointing your feet towards the teacher served as a mark of respect. You may be your own teacher, so let it become a habit to turn around, head nearest the mirror, and let your highest point reflect back at you.

STARTING POSITION: *top of the mat towards the mirror; lying with feet away from the mirror.*

SETTING UP Begin by lying back on your mat. Extend your arms on the floor at your sides, and place your feet under your knees.

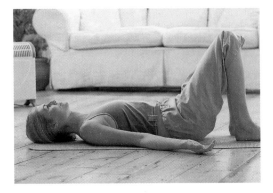

2 Relax the legs

Inhaling, slide your heels away and, pointing your toes evenly away from your ankles, gently stretch your legs. Exhaling, allow your legs gently to rotate away from the centre, hip socket to toes, and relax.

3 Position the head

Inhale and lift your head while keeping your shoulders in position; tuck your chin into your throat. Keep your chin tucked in as you replace the back of your head (prominent part of the skull). Exhale, allow the chin to lift to neutral and bring your face parallel to the floor. Your chin and forehead should be almost level.

1 Release the torso

Inhale and lift your hips and ribs. Begin to rotate the arms externally while rolling the shoulders back, then draw your shoulder blades together and down the spine. Exhale, and slowly lower your ribs one by one to the floor. The diamond space between your throat, navel and nipple line should feel open and relaxed. Just before your buttocks touch the floor, inhale and adjust your pelvis so that your belly and pelvic centre are aligned with the floor. If a full teacup were placed in the centre of your pelvic diamond (made by your navel, pubis and front hipbones), it would not spill. Exhale and set your buttocks on the floor without tilting; feel openness as you relax this area.

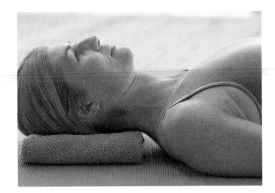

Hot tips Head drops back with the chin up high? Place a folded towel beneath your head to align your head and neck with the rest of your spine.

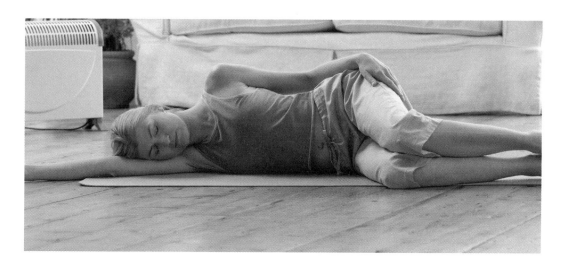

4 Turn inward

Softly close your eyelids and turn your gaze upwards and inward. Bring your attention to your breath as you begin to scan your body. As you inhale, turn inward and gently expand while gathering any unwanted sensations or thoughts, then gently exhale and release them. Try to synchronise the movement of your breath with your desired intention to relax and release, and feel the results. Let your mind direct the action, and note the sensation as you synchronise thoughts, feelings and actions into one-pointed mindfulness on the breath. You might find that the ideas on page 37 help you sink into this relaxation and re-energizing of body, mind and spirit.

COMING TO When ready to get up, keep your eyes closed and slowly wiggle your fingers and toes. Gently stretch your skin with soft, full breaths. Inhaling, draw your knees to your chest and right arm overhead. Exhale and roll to the right, using the upper right arm as a pillow, stacking shoulders, hips and legs. Extend your left arm over your left hip for support. Lie here for a few breaths. Try to feel the breath as it travels in and out through the back of your nostrils.

Hot tips Lying on your right side promotes left-nostril dominance, which encourages relaxation. Adopt the coming-to position—a good quick relaxation—when you really can't give yourself adequate time in Savasana. But try not to make a habit of it.

RESOURCES

Below is a selected list of studios in the United Kingdom, Australia and New Zealand that teach Bikram-based hot yoga; there are many more than are listed here. Get online and find a studio near you.

UNITED KINGDOM

Bikram Yoga Bristol
First Floor, 38 High Street
Bristol BS1 2AW
www.bikramyogabristol.com

Bikram Yoga Edinburgh
13 Edina Place
Edinburgh EH7 5RN
www.bikramyogaedinburgh.com

Bikram Yoga Glasgow
1 Dowanside Lane
Glasgow G12 9BZ
www.bikramglasgow.com

Bikram Yoga Fleet
242-244 Fleet Road
Hampshire GU51 4BX
www.bikramyogafleet.co.uk

Bikram Yoga Leeds
The Core, Level 2, The Headrow
Leeds LS1 6JD
www.bikramyogaleeds.com

Bikram Yoga London
4 Beaufort Court, Admirals Way
London E14 9XL
www.bikramyogalondon.com

Hot Yoga Society
1A Magdalen Street
London SE1 2EN
www.hotyogasociety.com

Sohot Bikram Yoga
Threeways House, 40-44 Clipstone
Street, Bolsover Street Entrance
London W1W 5DW
www.sohotbikramyoga.co.uk

Urban Bikram
18-24 Shacklewell Lane
London E8 2EZ
www.urbanbikram.com

YogaVenue
2 Avenue Lane
Oxford OX4 1YF
www.yogavenue.co.uk

Bikram Yoga Manchester
51 Church Street
Manchester M4 1PD
www.bikramyogamanchester.co.uk

B Yoga
59 Friar Lane
Leicester LE1 5RB
www.bikramyogaleicester.co.uk

Yoga Hub
First Floor, 21 Old Hall Street
Liverpool L3 9BS
www.yogahubliverpool.co.uk

AUSTRALIA AND NEW ZEALAND

Bikram Yoga Darlinghurst
256 Crown Street
Darlinghurst, Sydney, NSW 2010
www.bikramyoga.net.au

Yoga in Daily Life Australia
206 Woodville Road
Merrylands, NSW 2160
www.yogaindailylife.org.au

Bikram Hot Yoga Fitzroy
24-26 Johnston Street
Fitzroy, Melbourne, VIC 3065
www.bikramyogafitzroy.com.au

Bikram Yoga Prahran
Level 1, 236 High Street
Prahran, Melbourne, VIC 3181
www.bikramyogaprahran.com.au

Yoga in Daily Life New Zealand
23 Jessie Street
Te Aro, Wellington,
New Zealand 6011
www.yogaindailylife.org.nz

Bikram Hot Yoga North Shore
2-7 Mercari Way,
Albany ANZ Centre, Albany,
Auckland, New Zealand 0632
www.bikramyoganz.co.nz

GLOSSARY

Abduction Moving away from the centre of the body, or moving apart.

Adduction Bringing in towards centre or across centre, or bringing together.

Distal joints Pertaining to the joints away from centre.

Extension Opening at the joint and lengthening.

External rotation Turning away from the front of the body.

Flexion Bending at the joint and closing.

Full rotation Circling.

Internal rotation Turning towards the front of the body.

Neuroglandular Relating to nervous and glandular tissue. Reconditioning, by optimising regulatory communication and function between the two systems.

Neuromuscular Relating to nervous and muscle tissue. Reconditioning, by optimising communication and function between the two systems.

THE POSES

ENGLISH

Standing deep breathing

Half-moon pose

Hands-to-feet pose

Awkward pose

Eagle pose

Standing head-to-knee pose

Standing bow pulling pose

Balancing stick

Standing separate leg stretching pose

Triangle Pose

Tree pose

Toe stand pose

Wind–removing pose

Cobra pose

Half-locust pose

Full locust pose

Bow pose

Fixed firm pose

Half-tortoise pose

Camel pose

Rabbit pose

Head-to-knee pose

Stretching pose

Spine twisting pose

Blowing in firm (hero) pose

Dead body pose

ASANAS

SANSKRIT

Pranayama

Ardha chandrasana

Padahastasana

Utkatasana

Garudasana (Bikram spelling: Garuasana)

Dandayamana-janushirasana

Dandayamana-dhanurasana

Tuladandasana

Dandayamana-bibhaktapada-paschimot-thanasana

Trikonasana (Bikram spelling: Trikanasana)

Tadasana vrkasana

Padangustasana

Pavanamuktasana

Bhujangasana

Salabhasana

Poorna-salabhasana

Dhanurasana

Supta vajrasana

Ardha-kurmasana

Ustrasana

Sasangasana

Janushirasana

Paschimotthanasana

Ardha-matsyendrasana

Kapalbhati in vajrasana

Savasana

INDEX